Rolling A Path:
My Own
Narcolepsy, Skateboarding,
Cataplexy & Lifestyle

ISBN-13: 978-0989991919

ISBN-10: 0989991911

(Narcoplexic)

Narcoplexic@Narcoplexic.com

Much Thanks to my Mother, first and foremost.

Thank You to my family and familia Nica,
to my close friends and also to my lost
and/or misplaced friends.

Thank You, to anyone who appreciates what I do
and to those who try to understand.

Note/s:

Know that I am not a doctor and am in no way trying to act as one. Some of the things which I go into in detail in the book may for you possibly involve some risk/s. Anything that you do attempt is '_at your own risk._' What I go into are things that have helped me get to where I am today, finding a general stability.

There may be a bit of seemingly random use of word combinations as well as odd grammar or wording/s... Specifically, when it comes to Narcolepsy, be it Narcolepsy with Cataplexy or Narcolepsy without Cataplexy, it can be lengthy to differentiate such, each and every time when necessary. At times I just use the word Narcolepsy, when Narcolepsy with Cataplexy is what I'm referring to. Generally, it should be clear and/or within context. Being that I live having Narcolepsy with Cataplexy, that is the perspective.

Strange Note/s:

Narcolepsy with Cataplexy is what it is.

We are what we eat.

All be it one, as one be it all.

We may know what we know, but there is only so much which we can actually know, that is, of what all there is to know.

Regardless of how much is known, there is more to be.

To have any perspective at all requires viewing multiple perspectives.

Think and rest -- before, during and after.

There are times that a step backwards is better than a step forwards, or any step/ping at all.

Use caution aggressively, but also use aggression cautiously.

Be conscious rather than unconscious.

There's a path out there for each one of us.

No two paths are the same and/or equal.

No path is (exactly) simple nor clear and/or (necessarily) apparent.

Each one must seek and work towards finding their own path, for it does exist.

Book Note/s:
This may be a sort of long book. I don't know. Maybe it's not? As a first, hopefully it is follow-able and coherent? Hopefully, something will ring and/or echo to those that make their way through it? Whether what I say within actually holds any sort of weight and/or quality to or for you, only you can decipher.

Basically, this was written in a few different sittings over the past 6 months or so. A lot of it is background and what I felt was necessary to fit in, what would be, if not included, possible gaps. Somehow, I ended up with three sections to the book. At one point after beginning it with no clear set idea of where I was going to end up, I did decide that I wanted to elaborate on Skateboarding with Cataplexy interfering. To get there, I went into my parents, infancy, childhood and more. There was a point when I decided that I wanted to attempt including some of the factual information that I've learned about Narcolepsy with Cataplexy, described in my own way. So, that happened and ended up as the beginning section of the book.

Then lastly and more recently, I've really been wanting to express in some detail the Lifestyle Adjustments which have really helped me get to where I currently am. The path I've taken.

It's been a handful of years since I was experiencing serious Cataplexy (5-20 times daily for some months). About two years ago I was still collapsing fairly frequently (be it, 3-6 times each couple of months). But today, I've collapsed once (a couple of months ago) in what is now nearing a year. I've been med free and will remain med free as long as I can manage to. If things get back to the point they were at, I'd be more likely to consider them. But I stubbornly resist. Yet, I've done a lot of research (not a topic nor mentioned in this book) into the meds currently used; and I have zero confidence in, nor desire for, any of them.

To be very blunt and upfront, I will say something here which may make a few of you cringe and/or even close the book: Cannabis has helped me in real ways over the years. (Moderation and responsibility are hugely relevant and always within my focus). The current wave of level-headed-ness (referring to the laws changing) is wonderful and long, long overdue. Unless you feel that alcohol, tobacco, coffee and chocolate should all be things that get a person locked up, then please don't hate on Cannabis. That will be the only mention of it which I'll be doing in this book.

Table of Contents:

Author Note/s

This book has various purposes, but the two main reasons are to offer my own personal methods of juggling the disease in the hopes that perhaps some other/s out there may read and benefit from it. Within it, I try to express some understanding into, what is (for me) my own Narcolepsy with Cataplexy.

The terminology is difficult and can be a bit confusing at times. There is Narcolepsy, there is Narcolepsy with Cataplexy, there is Narcolepsy without Cataplexy; there is also Idiopathic Hypersomnolance, which is similar in many ways but basically lacking a couple of the symptoms. Commonly when speaking, I use the words 'condition / disorder / syndrome / neurological / endocrine / disease.' Perhaps the word 'disease' to an extent actually reflects entirely the effects and/or the entirety of the symptoms of Narcolepsy with Cataplexy. The actual disease is described in a plethora of different ways as well. For instance, all of the following, unfortunately, are fitting to it: degenerative disease, autoimmune disease, hormonal disease, and sleep disorder. While at Mayo Clinic in Rochester, MN, I asked the sleep specialist doctor what the proper terminology is, mentioning all of the above words. His response was that they are all fitting.

There is so much misunderstanding out there around Narcolepsy, and especially Cataplexy. This can make life awfully painful as well as very difficult. Living with the condition, one can often feel almost entirely misunderstood in terms of people's responses to it and their attempts to give reason or explanation to it. It can be hard and seemingly impossible to attempt expressing certain things, because of commonly held perceptions or concepts of what the disease involves combined with general social expectations. To expect that any ordinary person can easily begin to understand it may be, and most definitely is, too much to ask. For those who do live with Narcolepsy (with or without Cataplexy), understanding it takes time; and one must have a desire, as well as interest, in learning about it.

It took me a long while, years, to actually accept the possibility of Narcolepsy. At age 28, it seemed so unlikely and out of place upon the first contemplation of whether it could be Narcolepsy. Yet the Cataplexy explanation and criteria for what Cataplexy is, was just too exact and fitting, mirroring exactly what I'd been experiencing for so long and in ways as far back as I can recall). The more that I dove into it, the clearer and more obvious it all became. The symptoms appeared clear and present, but only gradually. Getting a solid grasp of what each symptom is, took real observation and deep reflection upon the varying experiences of others (described in forums).

Much of what I discuss and describe is coming straight from the long journey of attempting to grasp, as best I could (and/or can, as I continue to always seek further understanding) of what Narcolepsy with Cataplexy is. And what that is, for me.

For years now I've spent vast amounts of time, hours/days/weeks/months, reading research articles and papers, interacting with people in online forums, diving into their own stories and experiences as well. Current and past research is frequently provided and also discussed on the forums. Discussing with the doctors, with whom I've been given time to discuss the disease in depth, has been good. The best and most thorough conversation I've had was with the sleep specialist doctor at Mayo Clinic in Rochester, MN. I've met a few other persons with Narcolepsy (some with and some without Cataplexy). I attended an event for Narcolepsy research that also involved a 'research update/contribution' discussion, where I had a brief discussion one-on-one with Dr. Emmanuel Mignot. He is the world's most renowned Narcolepsy doctor and the Director of the Stanford Center for Narcolepsy. I was engaged very much in the discussion, asking questions as well as offering my own opinion and experiences in response to others' questions.

I took part online in the FDA's fourth Patient Focused Drug Development Initiative which was in September of 2013. Narcolepsy was chosen and will be receiving more focus as well as financial funding and incentives from the FDA, in regards to drug research.

In October of 2013, I attended the 28th Annual Narcolepsy Network Conference in Atlanta, where I met other persons with Narcolepsy and displayed the book of illustrations I'd recently finished [*Expressions of my own Narcolepsy with Cataplexy: An onward roller coaster ride, it is..(2013)*]. I am thinking to try to attend the conference again, this year (2014) in Denver, CO. Perhaps I could do a discussion/presentation on Lifestyle Adjustments with questions and answers.?!

For me to not dive into certain past events from throughout my life would leave certain points and things that I attempt to say, vague and unclear. It is difficult for me to not be thorough; but it is, at the same time, difficult for me to feel that I've been thoroughly heard and/or understood. Perhaps such is just related to my own mannerism and/or interpretation, my perception of others? But I do hope that I am able to convey the points I am actually attempting to make, and that these points will be clear and noted, not misunderstood.

This is my first book of prose writing. My earlier book was mainly illustrations with a brief description, pertaining mainly to my own

Narcolepsy with Cataplexy. The organization here is a bit scattered, but maybe it works? There's a lot from the past and about me that I've left out of this book. We'll see where I end up going on the next project, whenever that begins?

Please, though, bear with me through this one. It is my first go at putting my actual words out there; and it may require some depth, to interpret...

1st Grasp

For around 5 years now, I've known of the disease (whether or not it is described or labeled as) Narcolepsy with Cataplexy. Earlier, though I did not know what it was, it had caused me much difficulty throughout my life and in a lot of ways. Yet it has also made my life more interesting and definitely has forced me to view the world in what may be a different and/or atypical way. 'Narcolepsy with Cataplexy' is very misunderstood and in my own mind is something that, unless you are very close to someone who lives with it and you have a very open mind, it is unlikely that you have a full understanding and grasp of. Even living with it, it remains very confusing and never something that is fully graspable and/or controllable.

Especially through hindsight, I've been able to see and note a lot about the disease -- reflecting back over the many years that I've lived with the disease, when it was unknown to me; thinking of the odd experiences I've had. as well as the effects the different symptoms and the meshing of them have had upon me. There is much to see, much to contemplate upon and dissect in different manners; for instance, gauging how Cataplexy required continual adjusting and/or contorting of psychological posturing, or maneuvering, to remain hidden and out of my own perception. That is to say, in other words, that I had to intentionally keep myself from acting and/or involving myself in certain activities or levels of activity. Specific examples would be: I could not be joking around regularly out and about or while standing, I could not bring someone a plate of food but instead had to tell them to get it themselves (due to risk of dropping the plate and/or collapsing), etc... There are so many examples that I could never even try to think of them all, because the effects of the symptoms can be and are so deep and become masked and/or mixed into the whole bag.

There is clearly no consistent pattern to Narcolepsy with Cataplexy, nor simple view of living with it.

One of the hugest sources of information came from reading likely thousands of forum posts. People with the disease are writing and having back and forth dialogue, discussing their own experiences with the disease and sharing their stories.

There clearly are no two cases which are exactly the same. The symptoms vary from one person to the next, as does each symptom as well, for each person who lives with the disease. There are so many aspects to even each symptom, which can have multiple degrees of variation. It is extremely hard to understand. Still, Narcolepsy with Cataplexy, unfortunately, remains an entirely incurable disease. Some do find benefits from the symptomatic medications available, and others (such as myself) do and/or have not.

Lifestyle Adjustments have done wonders for me.

Research / Discoveries

Over the past 15 years there have been major discoveries regarding the possible causes of the disease. Many universities and some drug companies are doing research currently into Narcolepsy with Cataplexy. It has recently been chosen as one of 20 diseases to be given FDA funding for further research, because of the noted need for better treatments as well as better awareness of the disease within both society and the medical realm (being doctors and specialists).

In 1999 there were two very important discoveries made, basically around the same time and basically discovering the same thing. This discovery completely opened the door to more discoveries and brought a real advancement to the understanding of Narcolepsy with Cataplexy. After a series of research studies on Narcoleptic dogs, a new neuropeptide was discovered, an important neuropeptide which is responsible for regulating the sleep/awake states and much, so much, more.

A neuropeptide can also be called a hormone or a neurotransmitter. Vigilance, mood, wakefulness, arousal, appetite (glucose and fat metabolism) and other very critical traits, to do with one's controllable and/or manageable abilities, are all related in terms of regulation to the neuropeptide.

The discovery was made in two different places by two different entities at more or less the same time, resulting in two different names for the same thing, the newly discovered neuropeptide. The two names are Orexin and Hypocretin.

There is both Orexin A (Hypocretin I) and Orexin B (Hypocretin II). Being Human Biology, it all gets very much more complicated. Orexin or Hypocretin plays within the endocrine system, which means there are some of the same neuron cells in the gut yet it is slightly different and referred to as Orexin B (Hypocretin II). Regardless, this neuropeptide Orexin A (Hypocretin I) is only found in small quantities within the brain's spinal cord, the hippocampus and the hypothalamus (where it is, or should be, produced). What was discovered to be perhaps the main cause of the disease in the Narcoleptic dog study was that the Orexin (Hypocretin) was missing, and entirely so in those with Cataplexy. Humans and mice were then tested through spinal tap measurements of their Orexin (Hypocretin) levels; and the discovery was made that humans who have Narcolepsy with Cataplexy have low levels to no levels of Orexin (Hypocretin) in their brain.

It was a hugely important discovery, and today it has become apparent that there is an auto immune system process or element to Narcolepsy with Cataplexy. The cells (neuropeptides) get killed off for some reason, relating to an auto immune system response. More recently, it has been discovered that persons with Narcolepsy have very high levels of another neuropeptide, that being specifically Histamine (related to allergies). Currently, the hypothesis is that perhaps the excess histamine cells are killing off the Orexin/Hypocretin cells, thus possibly being the biologic cause of Narcolepsy.

As far as genetics goes, there is a common human leukocyte antigen (HLA) marker found in the blood, which can indicate a greater likelihood of one developing Narcolepsy, though having this marker (**HLA-DQB1*0602**) does not mean that you will develop the disease. Around 90% of people that have Narcolepsy will test positive for the marker. Something like 20% of the general population will test positive for this marker, while only between 1 in 2,000 to 3,000 persons have Narcolepsy, according to the Stanford

Center for Narcolepsy.

Other discoveries which have been made, have to do with certain illnesses triggering the loss of Orexin/Hypocretin, therefore causing Narcolepsy. A few of the illnesses, which have been tied to such killing off of the cells, are strep throat and certain flu viruses.

In recent years in Europe, there has been a large law suit after thousands of cases were diagnosed of childhood Narcolepsy occurring in children who were given a rushed monovalent 2009 H1N1 influenza vaccine (made by Pandremix).

The Diagnosis

There is no single test currently, nor is one likely to be developed, that will 100% specifically test for Narcolepsy.

Currently, the Multiple Sleep Latency Test (MSLT) is the main testing method for Narcolepsy. Sleep latency refers to the amount of time it takes you to fall asleep and into rapid eye movement (REM).   Before you start the test, you have to fill out a sleep questionnaire. They then begin gluing about 30 nodes, mostly on your head, to read your brain waves for the electroencephalogram (EEG). They video monitor you overnight and speak to you through an intercom. They put a pulse oxymeter on your finger to read your blood oxygen saturation levels overnight (which relates directly to checking for sleep apneas).   The MSLT measures how quickly (within how many minutes) and how often the patient falls asleep and into Rapid Eye Movement (REM). The MSLT generally follows after a polysomnography (sleep study) and consists of the patient taking a series of 4 or 5 short, 15-20 minute, naps throughout a day. After each nap, the technician comes in and asks about whether or not you dreamed, asking you to write a description of the dreams that you had. If a patient has a sleep latency averaging below 8 minutes and the patient also has 2 sleep-onset REM periods (called SOREMPs), the diagnosis of Narcolepsy will be made.

The MSLT is not the most consistent test and more often than not people have to take it multiple times.

There are current possibilities of a blood test for Narcolepsy becoming available, at some point. Something was discovered to do with auto reactive T-cells?

Cataplexy is a unique symptom of Narcolepsy. If a patient has clear-cut Cataplexy (being the patient collapses from the common triggers like laughing, remaining conscious and able to hear as well as see), sometimes the diagnosis is made by the doctor without an

MSLT occurring.

The diagnosis criteria though can be quite strict. The diagnosis can also be quite difficult to reach, if, for instance (like occurred with me), the patient during their polysomnography appears to have any type of sleep apnea.

Sleep apnea is very complicated as well. We're talking sleep disorders, so that to me means things that are very unknown and/or possibly unknowable. Sleep apnea (know, there are many varying types) can often be confusable with Narcolepsy, because of excessive daytime sleepiness (EDS) being a main symptom. Determination comes down to sleep patterns and reading these is no simple task; but there can be clear distinctions which separate the sleep disorders. Expertise really is required to achieve proper confirmations.

What happens if the person does turn out to have sleep apnea during the first overnight polysomnography? The MSLT will be delayed until the sleep apnea is treated. This creates all sort of trickery and difficulties with regards to insurance approvals and acceptances...

Idiopathic Hypersomnolence is diagnosed when a person doesn't have Cataplexy, along with when they don't have SOREMP's during the MSLT but still have a sleep latency mean below the 8 minute guidelines. It is becoming more and more a part of the Narcolepsy community. At the Narcolepsy Network Conference, there were many people who have Idiopathic Hypersomnolence attending. They were curious about many of the same questions being asked by the persons who have Narcolepsy. Many persons get different diagnoses between the two diseases, by different doctors as well as by the same doctor at different points over time.

Narcolepsy is considered a *hyper*somnia to this day by the authors of medical text books, even though it is in combination with *hypo*somnia in a continually variable back and forth, because you both cannot sleep well and also cannot stay awake.

For me, such began a long and difficult as well as painful road (which I'll go into further, later within) to the diagnosis that I received at Mayo Clinic, 'Probable Narcolepsy with Cataplexy' with clear-cut Cataplexy. The 'Probable' was due to my sleep latency average being 9 minutes, 1 minute above the guideline cutoff of 8 minutes for the sleep latency mean. Also, it was agreed that the door to the room that I was sleeping in, being opened, a few minutes into my 3rd nap, skewed the test; likely having raised the sleep latency mean.

The 4 Tetrad Symptoms of Narcolepsy

The four main [tetrad] symptoms of Narcolepsy are the following:

1) *Excessive Daytime Sleepiness (EDS)*
2) *Hypnagogic Hallucinations*
3) *Sleep Paralysis*
4) *Cataplexy*.

1) -*Excessive Daytime Sleepiness (EDS)*-: is being very tired, to the point that it is affecting you. You may be yawning frequently and even nodding off, falling asleep or day dreaming uncontrollably. For me it can be a physical fatigue, the physical body having become so tired that it aches and is difficult, at times, to continue walking and/or to continue standing up straight. There can be a mental fog or cloud, which is like having a web or net wrapped around your thoughts. Thinking and focusing, concentrating what so ever, is beyond difficult. At times, fighting hard with the physical body to attempt at awakening (trying to focus) the mental strength, and at other times, you fight so hard with the mental strength (focusing on physical strength) to continue moving with the physical body. For me it means awakening after sleeping for what should be for the average person a full night's rest (consisting of 7 or 8 hours sleep), feeling more tired than when you'd gotten into bed to go to sleep the night prior. Or it can mean at times, within an hour of awakening, being struck by what feels like a wall of bricks, of lethargy/tiredness/weakness. It varies, causing different effects a lot of the time; and it is unpredictable, sometimes even quite un-note-able (in that dull cloud, so to speak, mentally and physically).

What I've learned and managed to do to better myself with regards to the EDS, since discovering that I have Narcolepsy, has not been easy. But, I have found a few things which have helped me overall. They are not necessarily simple things though. They all have to do with Lifestyle Adjustments, which I'll be going more into depth on later within.

Within the Narcolepsy community (as the forums participants refer to themselves) there are words used, like 'micro-sleeps' and 'sleep attacks.' These words are commonly used to describe a couple of different variations of occurrences. To try to explain them, I'll just describe 'micro-sleeps' as when you find yourself daydreaming (actually having dreams while awake) while continuing on with whatever activity that you are doing. This may also be described, to an extent, as 'Automatic Behavior' in other circumstances or situations. I'll describe 'sleep attacks' as being an occurrence of extreme tiredness overtaking you, being so tired all of a sudden that you can no longer think nor even focus. It is not falling asleep mid-sentence, but it is like all of a sudden being drugged to the point that you must sleep. A term I tend to use, is 'nodding off' and it is to mean exactly that: my head begins to feel heavy and my mind has begun dreaming, I am going in and out of REM dreaming and being awake, trying to retain any focus or mental capacity. This happens to me semi-frequently in the evening, if I am unable to keep myself stimulated by something of interest or by doing some physical activity, if I have the strength for it. This symptom alone has made a severe impact on my ability to work because, unless I am doing something that I am both interested in and to an extent enjoying, there is nothing I can do to prevent the 'nodding off' from occurring nor stop it once it has begun. Snapping out of it can be difficult because it creeps right back.

2) -*Hypnagogic Hallucinations (Dreams)*-: vivid and intense, dreams which can be of very familiar or obscure situations, sometimes auditory but always visually intense and/or confusing. These are something that one has difficulty with at times, because they can leave a person scared and baffled as well as deeply confused. They occur typically as one is falling asleep or as one is awakening from sleep, somewhere in between the different sleep stages.

For me, these have definitely left me very uneasy, and during them very frightened, tense and out right scared. They've involved no specific person that I know; but unknown figures and the environment that I am sleeping within are definite common factors of these odd dreams/hallucinations.

During one of these episodes I may, for instance, be hearing something like an accident occurring outside, then actually be thinking that I'm awake in the bed, noting flashing red and blue lights along with hearing sirens, all coming from outside of my window, then hearing a series of voices and chatting or bickering, and then a loud pounding knock on the door with a yelling voice, demanding that I open the door. But then I was stuck frozen, frightened and unable to move, gradually falling back into sleep (though, in fact, I was mainly asleep the entire time). The following morning I was somewhat confused. The first thing I did was look out my front window and at my door, just to see whether there were any remnants of a car accident or something to note. There was nothing, and I also asked my Mother whether she'd heard or noted anything during the night prior, which she said that she'd not.

Another instance was having gotten into my bed without turning off the light of my room (it was one of those uncontrolled sleepiness moments when I go from the chair right into the bed). Suddenly in bed, I noted that there was an odd aura or presence in the room and I gradually tried glancing in the other direction. As I did so, I noted a couple of odd figures nearing me, but especially the faces are what I noted, because they were not exactly viewable in the light. As the faces got closer to me, they appeared like small clouds of smoke in a gray and/or yellow shade. During this, I began to awaken (for real) and in my mind I remembered the word 'hypnagogic.' At the same moment I made the effort to open my eyes. As my eyelid opened, I noted that I was completely safe and comfortably in my room. I also noted that the faces dissipated and the smoke and figures (puff) cleared away. What was sort of amazing to me about this occurrence was that I let myself go right back to sleep, immediately closing my eyes again. This was likely because of how comfortable I was, in that I could remember this was just a symptom of Narcolepsy; and I recognized/knew my place, from having slightly opened my eye/s. As I fell right back into sleep, the faces reappeared, so I did the same. It went in and out, a few more times, sort of playing with it, and was left with an odd experience in the end, which I actually sort of enjoyed.

It would shock me if these hypnagogic hallucinations (dreams) are not something that each and every person experiences at some point of their life, if not on multiple and random occasions. There is definitely something, like also with Cataplexy, that relates directly to a person's stress and anxiety levels. What I'm saying there is that when one is awfully stressed or is very anxious, perhaps about some upcoming event, the chances and likelihood of a hypnagogic hallucination (dream) occurring goes way up.
The only times that these seem to happen to me are around times

when I have been very stressed out, perhaps bothered and/or disgruntled from some interaction or occurrence, or when I have some upcoming activity or pressure upon me. During such times, I actually have begun to basically expect these to occur. A common time I seem to have these is before traveling, with the anxiousness and knowing I'll have to awaken at a specific time. Perhaps they occur on such occasions because I frequently throughout my sleep am thinking of having to awaken at a specific time and/or am concerned about not oversleeping or whatever is involved the following morning/day. Thus, limiting how deep or light I can sleep, sort of tangling up or twisting up the sleep stages which (perhaps sometimes) are of a more natural routine/process? Maybe sleep apnea triggers them on an occasion?

Another thing about these hypnagogic hallucinations (dreams) is that they can potentially be so realistic and involved, including real persons as well as activities from one's daily life. They can actually confuse a person into thinking that certain things have occurred. Thankfully, I've not had trouble with this and have been able to decipher quite simply between when something has been a dream and when things are concretely real. But, I'd be lying to say that there's not been a couple of times when dreams depicting times from my childhood left me a bit baffled and momentarily confused for a while. That is all only in terms, though, of reflecting upon past occurrences and nothing that is grave or questionable. There has been an occurrence or two, of my asking a friend about something that lingered from a dream, and them simply being like 'what?' which at that point confirmed for me that whatever it was, was in a dream...

3) -*Sleep Paralysis*-: Awake, yet paralyzed. It is exactly that, like Cataplexy in the aspect that when one is dreaming there is muscle

atonia (a paralysis of the muscles) to prevent one from enacting their dream/s. Sleep paralysis is a lingering sort of effect, in that one actually awakens but their body does not (yet) as the atonia remains.

This can be frightening for persons to experience, and it is often something which combines with hypnagogic hallucinations (dreams), increasing their intensity because you cannot react, move, nor run.

Sleep paralysis is the one symptom that I think I've experienced the least, of the 4 tetrad symptoms of Narcolepsy. The experiences I've had with it have been wrapped up in or with experiences of hypnagogic hallucinations (dreams) where I've been too frightened to move (yet, in a weird way sometimes I'm not really frightened but rather just frozen, nervous, and tense).

Sleep paralysis may also be something that occurs in a less grave manner at times. This is to say that it can be possible to move slightly but not entirely, making waking up and arising from bed extremely difficult. This condition is, I believe, still considered 'sleep paralysis' within the medical definitions or understandings. Definitely, I can remember having serious difficulty in awakening, feeling as though my body was concrete and nearly impossible to move. It would take every available bit of strength and possible effort (both mentally and physically) to make movements to rise out of bed. The effect remains for a while, too, gradually dissipating.

4) -*Cataplexy*-: ranges from a minimal loss of muscle tone to complete temporary muscle paralysis, triggered by emotional inter-activity that is related to pleasure/s, triggers that are most often pleasurable engagements such as laughing.

Cataplexy can be as minimal as a slight facial spasm or a slight drooping of the head. Often 'a buckling of the knee/s' is described. It can also be as severe as being temporarily completely muscularly paralyzed. In fact, some persons who have Narcolepsy with Cataplexy during severe attacks/episodes can fall into sleep and not awaken for minutes to even hours. There are stories of people who have awoken in morgues...

During Cataplexy episodes/attacks, where the person is entirely paralyzed, the 'autonomous system' kicks in, and breathing as well as vital signs like the pulse are 'automatic.' Yet, like when one is asleep, breathing appears very light and/or shallow, being perhaps hard to note.

Cataplexy is a unique symptom to Narcolepsy. The closest thing to which it may be similar to, is epileptic seizures. Although, in contrast to epilepsy, when one experiences a Cataplexy attack/episode (as I will term it) they remain fully conscious throughout it, able to think, to hear and often also to see (depending to an extent upon the person and the intensity of the attack, and the position the person may end up in).

Cataplexy is described as 'an intrusion of the REM (rapid eye movement) sleep stage upon the waken state.' This is more or less to say that during sleep, when one is in a deep dream state (being the REM sleep stage), their body is physically paralyzed due to the muscle atonia which is a natural effort by the body to keep one from enacting their dreams in their sleep. The intrusion of REM into the waken state is triggered by the emotions. The person experiences muscle atonia, ranging from perhaps being slightly weak in the neck and drooping their head forwards, all the way to perhaps immediately collapsing awkwardly to the ground, paralyzed.

During more severe Cataplexy attacks/episodes (being when one collapses and is entirely unable to move) the person has no reflexes and the body is entirely limp.

It is said that as long as the person experiencing the Cataplexy does not injure themselves during the attack/episode, there is 'no harm' from Cataplexy. Injury may result, for example, from falling and/or an obstructing of their breathing somehow due to the position the person ended up in from the attack/episode.

Not all persons with Narcolepsy experience Cataplexy; and it is very, very rare for someone to have 'Idiopathic Cataplexy' or Cataplexy without Narcolepsy. Cataplexy without Narcolepsy is possible in neurological disease or spinal cord injuries, but it is not something you can easily find much actual information on.

To go into more depth on my own Cataplexy.
As a child, when I was tickled intensely and especially in the belly, my arms would go entirely limp and I could not move them what-so-ever. This seemed odd, but being able to roll around and continue to laugh out loud, stating that "I can not stop you, my arms won't move" which only seemed to bring on more tickles...
Later in life, Cataplexy triggers for me became things like joking around or trying to tell a joke to others; doing something kind and feeling joy in the interaction or exchange; receiving compliments; or any unanticipated or unexpected occurrence/interaction, such as smiles, silliness, being confronted suddenly, having intense frustration or anger, etc...
It is all complex and variable. Regarding the triggers or triggering of Cataplexy, there are endless ends (being no rules nor real consistency) as to how come, why, when, what, whom, or where...

Cataplexy is triggered during random and most often unpredictable interactions which do involve heightened emotion/s. Sometimes there is a somewhat predictable likelihood and sensing of an on-coming occurrence. A person who has Narcolepsy with Cataplexy will know that Cataplexy is going to hit, but not know when. For the person who has Narcolepsy with Cataplexy, there is neither a rule book nor a text book. Cataplexy is unpredictable and is, or can be, a real burden. It can create (or open up) real limitations and potential dangers for the person with it.

In my own opinion from my own experience with Cataplexy, one can do a lot to control it or have some sense to/of when it may occur, but that is only to a point. If you know your own boundaries well and can remain within them, Cataplexy can be less intense and/or less likely to occur. This very much involves for me, every aspect of life, including nearly complete detachment from involvement with all but a few people. This, I think, is what is described as isolation, mentioned in regards to Narcolepsy. This lifestyle is not easy and is, or can be, quite impact-full upon one's life in a negative way. Choosing to refrain from certain activity or activities can simply put, rule out the potential likelihood of Cataplexy occurring, or having to experience some ordeal around it.

For instance, I choose to continue skateboarding now and then, even though at times Cataplexy interferes. Perhaps my facial expression will be goofy as a brief sensation of a wave flows through my face, or maybe I'll have a flicker or momentary flinch of my upper body while skateboarding. Only once did I completely collapse from Cataplexy while skateboarding, due to the exhaustion and pleasure of landing the trick I was in the process of landing.

'Cataplexy with Narcolepsy?'

In my own mind, due to the manner in which I lived for so long, entirely unaware of the 'Narcolepsy' for what it was, it almost feels more fitting to describe my own case as 'Cataplexy with Narcolepsy.' In many ways the Cataplexy has impacted my life in more ways and restricted my ability in certain behaviors and/or activities, than the Narcolepsy. At the same time, the two (Narcolepsy and Cataplexy) do fit together. The effects of living with Narcolepsy, which include a continual and/or frequent lack of restorative sleep (simply a broken sleep pattern), may have resulted over time in my developing Cataplexy and/or having escalated events of Cataplexy.

It is important to mention how confusing and variable as well as difficult it is to actually understand the different symptoms of Narcolepsy, especially the vast variations in how each symptom can present itself. It's all hard to grasp. This disease has a history of being misunderstood, misdiagnosed and misrepresented, I think for a reason. Narcolepsy, obviously, does not mean falling asleep or being tired. Cataplexy is the odd symptom of Narcolepsy. It has all been portrayed most often in society by media and in film as falling asleep, suddenly and/or awkwardly.

There are countless forum post/s by persons with Narcolepsy who describe that it took reading others' experiences and stories, taking in others' feelings and reflections upon their own long processes of grasping, recognizing and being diagnosed with Narcolepsy (as was the process for me as well). On top of that, for me it took a long time involving difficult interactions and tests. Lots of confusion and unknowns...

To finally get the confirmation and grasp of what Narcolepsy with Cataplexy is, to recognize my own disease and to learn my own boundaries and limitations with regards to the symptoms variable affects has been quite relieving. If it weren't for my Mother, to whom I owe everything, the limitations and I don't know what that I'd be deep in, would be way over my head.

Frequently, I reflect upon this and it is a very scary thing to look at for the future, but at the exact same time, it is a fortunate thing. What I can do, I do, and I think her not being alone is a good thing. We definitely eat well, which is beneficial all-around and is one of the biggest adjustments I've made and am continuing to maintain as time goes on...

Parents / Family / Familia

My Mother is someone with an enormous heart, who has taught me the most, and especially how both to see the world as well as how to care about people. She has a PhD in Folklore Librarian Studies (something along those lines) and she works endlessly. Her passion which she enjoys is to work hard. She is in her mid-sixties currently and remains working full time, often doing work at home during her time off (thankfully, nothing like she'd been doing a few years back, where it was nearly every moment on or off from work). She has an aerobics class which she does for 1 hour, 3 times a week; and she goes walking with her friend and her friend's dog nearly every day. She insists on mowing the lawn and I find her doing mundane tasks around the house often. I do occasionally mow the lawn; and I do help with the tasks around the house, as much as possible.

My Father is someone who has a passion for music and especially music history. He has a PhD in Music History. He plays piano and the organ. For years I lost touch with him; in part or in many ways, I think that is because we are very similar and it was likely easier for us both. However, at a point after many years, I had to track him down because it seemed not right having lost touch for so long. It would not surprise me in the least, if he also has the disease Narcolepsy. His manner of being passionate about what he loves is something that I see in myself.

My one brother is 6 years older than me. He is awesome, very smart and is a hard worker. He does what he enjoys. He has taught me a lot through simply being a very good role model, as far back as I can recall. After graduating high school he gave me my first computer, which was a gateway to what became a real interest for me. He was building computers back in the late 80's and is an engineer, as well as many other things. We get along very well. We don't talk a whole lot, but we do keep in touch and visit on occasions. I've got mad respect for my brother.

My step Father is Nicaraguan, and lives a majority of the time in Managua still. My Mother married him in 1993. El Panson, I call him and he calls me, it means big bellied or pregnant (he was pretty large when I first met him and somehow the word stuck, to this day). He is a fun, caring and smart guy, who has been through a lot (as has any Nicaraguan). He makes my Mother really happy and reminds me of her in his devotion to what he does (education related) in Nicaragua.
Hopefully he will retire and move here one day before too long, which would make her super happy.
It would also perhaps help me feel better about any potential moving away, if ever possible by whatever opportunity?

Who I consider my Familia Nica is the family of the household where I spent many weeks and months over the years. They are incredible people who care a lot, more than almost any others that I've known. They taught me countless things of value, meaning and importance. It's a different world that they live in down there, and one that is super friendly, yet difficult in so many ways.

Infancy

The first six months of my life were an intense ride, which thankfully I don't remember for the obvious reason. But it was somehow similar to what I experienced later in life over the course of a few years, as I attempted to find help from doctors and within the medical realm (as I call it).

At 2 months old, I began to have severe seizures. I would begin to turn purple and then convulse. The first time it happened, my parents rushed me to the pediatrician's office, where I had a second seizure in front of the doctor, who then had my parents take me straight to the hospital, where I had a series of tests. After that my Mother slept with her hand on my back, so that if I had a seizure in the night, she could run with me to the hospital (which is two blocks from the house). I was put on medications for epilepsy at the time. Over the next two months I was seen by a local neurologist. The seizures continued to occur and the doctors told my parents over and over that "your son appears to be a perfectly healthy baby, except for the epileptic seizures he is having." My parents became frustrated because the seizures were continuing to occur and were becoming more frequent, more severe and lasting longer. Upon advice from a friend who felt her son's life had been saved by Mayo Clinic, my parents asked our local neurologist to get me into Mayo Clinic, and he set up an appointment for ten days hence at the Clinic. Feeling it was more urgent, my parents decided to rush to Mayo Clinic and to sit in the waiting room at St. Mary's Hospital (the Mayo Clinic hospital) until I turned purple (which happened many times each day) and then ask for me to be admitted. This was around a 17 hour drive. Upon our arrival my parents were shocked to learn that their friend (not our doctor) had arranged to have admission papers waiting, and I was immediately admitted. Within 24 hours of arriving at the emergency room in Rochester,

MN, it was determined that I had 'severe hyperinsulinemia hypoglycemia.' My pancreas had an over-supply of insulin-producing islets, resulting in extremely low blood sugar that caused the seizures to occur. So, after about 10 days of pediatric endocrinologists at Mayo Clinic monitoring me in the hospital, two options were described to my parents. One involved a night-time feeding tube and a diet regiment; the other was a surgery as delicate as open-heart surgery to remove about 95% or more of my pancreas in hopes of normalizing my insulin levels. After days of testing, the doctors decided I was a candidate for the surgery. It thankfully went well. I was then 4 months old. The strings it involved were, five years of 'blood sugar' monitoring along with taking an insulin-suppressing drug called Diazoxide' (because my insulin levels were still high for my body weight) and having follow up visits, which were part of a study being done at the time. As I grew, my pancreas adjusted to my body weight and I no longer needed the Diazoxide. They warned my parents that I was at a high risk of developing diabetes some day in my lifetime and that I also had a smaller risk of developing epilepsy in the future. Fortunately, I have never had another epileptic seizure nor do I have diabetes.

My parents have mentioned that as an infant sometimes while they'd be tickling me or making me smile, that I would all of a sudden stop reacting and go limp, losing my smile and/or facial expression. At the time, they thought I was stopping enjoying the playing, and they would stop. This was something they mentioned not long after discovering what Cataplexy was and having a better understanding of it.

Childhood / Teenage / 20's, Health

The first 5 years of my life I grew up taking an odd metallic medication and having my fingers pricked for 'blood sugar' testing a few times daily.

Around age 4, my dentist discovered that I had two large 'denticianist cysts' growing in my mouth, and a surgery was done to remove them. Throughout my life I've had dental matters come and go. One tooth required four root canal treatments (root canal retreat and others) before finally I decided this year to have it pulled. This was after, out of nowhere, it began hurting severely. There clearly was some fault of my own for the teeth matters I experienced earlier on in my life, since a teenager I did drink a whole lot of soda.

Around age 6, I began to have ear infections frequently, which to this day still occur. In fact, after age 6, when I had the first (of three sets of) 'myringetomy tubes' put into my eardrums, I've been unable to swim or, I should say, dip my ears into water. That was and remains unfortunate. My brother, who was six years older than me, swam competitively from about third grade through high school. I was also swimming regularly up until around age of 6 or 7, when I was told to stop by the ENT. To this day, if I get water in my ears, I will get a prompt ear infection which is painful and debilitating, so...

In elementary school I began experiencing severe and debilitating headaches and migraines. One of the teachers (from 4th to 6th grades) told my parents that they'd never seen a child have such severe headaches. The headaches continue, although thankfully not as often and also not normally as severe, compared to how they'd been throughout my childhood and my teens. Throughout all of my schooling years and through college as well, this is also an aspect of why I've had difficulty in ever working full time. I missed on average at least one day of school a week. In middle school on my way home on the bus one day, I vomited all over the seat in front of me due to a bad headache. In high school on a school trip in a van, I demanded they stop immediately, as I had to jump out vigorously and proceed to vomit (I remember having built up force as I began) due to a bad headache.

Today, as I mentioned, the headaches are less often and less severe. This has been only possible with much juggling of many 'lifestyle factors' which I've managed to tune.

At around 13 years old, I went back to the Mayo Clinic in Rochester, MN, and was examined and tested by an endocrinologist. Everything appeared to be normal and I was given a thumbs-up in terms of my pancreas, at least. This was the last time I was seen in regards to my original health matters. When I was there in 2011, nothing was said or done in regards to the pancreas.

Throughout my late teens and my 20's I was experiencing all sorts of frequent nose and throat problems. It was hard for me to even pick up on it though, as I was also experiencing frequent and near constant fatigue.

Throughout childhood and especially during high school, I was an athlete, playing ice hockey in the winters and Skateboarding nearly daily for hours most all of the years.

For so many years I'd managed to battle and fight through whatever ailments I was dealing with, in a way thinking that much of it was 'normal.' (Quick note: I do not like the word 'normal' and I try to use it somewhat cautiously.)

Everyone gets tired. Most people get headaches, dental matters or ear infections now and then. Everyone will get the flu and/or a cough now and then. These matters, that I had so often, were just things that I'd become quite used to and couldn't avoid or do much of anything about (so it seemed). Any time I take off my shirt and look at my belly, there is an 8" scar which reminds me of my pancreas. I'd grown up knowing my health was, in ways, at risk and that from the beginning some things had been, not well. This sort of conditioned me, I think, to be somewhat reserved and/or conscious, at least, that perhaps my lifetime would be shorter than the average person's, knowing that 90-95%+ of my pancreas had been removed and that at such an age, in infancy, my belly had been cut open, not to mention the trauma and drama of having the multiple severe seizures. In many respects, I am sure there are still lingering sorts of 'Post Traumatic Stress Disorder' (PTSD) effects from it all...

College

Starting the semester after finishing high school, I went directly into college. I had no specific major nor real specific interest in mind. Career wise, I did not know what I wanted or would be able to do. However, 'General Studies' was basically in the back of my mind as what to go towards. Going to college was something my parents had expected of me. With their help in applying early for Pell grants, along with my Mother working at the university in my hometown, tuition was covered; and I actually received a bit of cash each semester. Considering I stayed living at home, with the college being in the same city, there were no major moves or ordeals. During the first semester though, there was a massive hurricane that hit a part of Nicaragua that I was very familiar with. In fact, Nicaragua is and especially then was, my 2nd home. Growing up, between ages 8 and 22, I spent weeks to a month or two each year visiting a household in Nicaragua, in a small village which is very much like stepping into centuries past in terms of living conditions. It was 1998 and Hurricane Mitch caused a devastating mudslide near the village, killing over 2,000 people. Because of my close ties with the people there and my Mother's involvement in a Sister Cities Organization with my hometown and the village in Nicaragua, a 'relief aid' trip was planned, and I gathered three friends, who were each interested in helping. We four joined a 'Pastors for Peace' caravan driving through Central America. So, in December of 1998 I dropped my classes, making the proper arrangements and departed on a trip, driving to the village affected by the mudslide in Nicaragua. The trip took three weeks of driving and was very intense at times, but is something that I learned a lot by doing and also is something that I will never forget. Upon returning, I immediately enrolled back in school and was in classes in January.

By the 3rd semester in college, I'd decided that I was interested in learning as much about computers as I could, unfortunately computer hardware/technician sorts of classes and/or degrees, were not something the university offered. But, I did take a lot of different sorts of basic computer software classes with a couple network hardware classes which gave me a very solid grasp on using many different programs. It also helped to be able to understand generally and very well how and what makes computers function, along with computer networking. It took me until 2003 to finish and receive my Bachelor's in General Studies with a focus on computer science.

Throughout college there was a sort of heaviness, a fog or cloud that I fought through. It is hard to describe. But when you are tired, it can be hard to think and focus. To concentrate requires extra effort. You become dull and the tiredness can become disguised. This was what I experienced every single day. And I should say I can still experience this when I am really exhausted, possibly combined with being rushed and/or being pressured. There were massive amounts of stress and also anxieties during college, with the due dates and what not. In addition, there were many bouts of depression, some of which were very dark. I can remember really bumming some of my good friends out with my matters. At that point in time, I was completely aware of both the depression and something else with my health being off. But I had no recognition as to what it was that was off, and I had no idea that I was really, really tired.
The depression I recognized and fought battles with, until finally I got to a point where it was just maybe there occasionally. I've benefited from the experiences I've had living in Nicaragua, the 3rd world living conditions and general focus there, which is just so

different than what is common here in the 1st world. Usually, through some simple reflecting, depression for me can be overcome. Not always easily though.

Each night I would sleep like a rock and I would sleep at least 8 to 10, sometimes 12 or 13 hours. This was in part by choice and because I could. During these years I gradually cut down on the amount of soda that I was drinking, until around age 23 or 24, I completely cut it out. Each and every day, I was eating out, not fast food so much, but eating lunch and/or dinner at the nice restaurants around town. Where I live there are many types of ethnic restaurants and at lunch many have buffets. Indian food was one of the favorites to eat, Mexican was another favorite, but the Indian food was most frequent. From one friend to a handful of friends would meet up for lunch throughout the weeks, randomly. Between ages 18 and 23, I'd gained 60 to 70 pounds, around age 24 in 2004, I weighed close to 250 pounds, possibly more.

¿Health & Depression?

Before age 20, I knew that there was more to my health; I knew that something was 'not normal.'

For years and years, I just could not help but wonder what it was that was underlying my health matters, but the thought of attempting to explain it to a doctor was heavy and uncomfortable. Not even being able to specifically explain it to myself, there was no way I'd be able to explain it all to a doctor. The details were so clouded, as far as what to specifically say, and how to say whatever I would say.

Having attempted to get help with my headache and migraine problems, in the past, I'd gotten nowhere on numerous attempts. Having attempted to get help in regards to odd sensations with my hands and arms, which were said to be a Neuropathy or Carpal Tunnel Syndrome, such had also gotten nowhere beyond learning the terms.

The pancreas was always in the back of my mind, but Mayo Clinic had told me it was just fine.

From about 18 on, I'd been experiencing a sort of lethargic fatigue, and way too often, really, every single day. I'd become so used to it, that I didn't hardly recognize it for what it was, as I basically mentally thrived (painfully) through everything that I had to get through. Depression mounted and grew over time, yet I'd manage to release it somehow by sleeping as much as I could (unknowing as to how much it all related to sleep).

It had been years and years, since my teens, that I'd been experiencing bouts of depression, and at times in a bad way; yet it was always entirely recognizable. I was conscious of being depressed and managed to remain more or less stable.

Again, the travels I'd done visiting Nicaragua, a 3rd World country, had taught me a lot about being grounded, recognizing and appreciating the things which we in the 1st World should be thankful and respectful for having. Things really for me have been wonderful. My life has been beautiful in so many ways and I've been gifted to experience so much. For me, what really helps when I'm struggling combat the depression is to take a step backwards in the mind: a reflection upon the larger picture of the world which is outside of one's self; thinking of that which is elsewhere being, rather, in my place; putting into my perspective another from a place that is different from my own. Sometimes the reflections that occur are real and fascinating. The happiness and kindness of persons who live in conditions which seem ancient is incredible. There are trade-offs, everywhere and within everything.

That is all, which is not to say that I don't still experience depression or feeling down and/or bitter, because it would be a lie to say that I do not.

Viewpoint / Opinion

The truth is, in my own mind, that we live in a fascinating and miraculous time, a time period full of things which could not have even been considered a century ago.

I love to observe. I love to contemplate. I love learning and taking in all that I can. I love reflecting. I love nature.

And as much as it is difficult for me to feel that I can nearly ever in any way be understood, I do love attempting to understand things. At the same time, I definitely also feel and recognize that only so much can actually ever be understood, that a large part of living this life is acknowledging that there are things which are not meant to be understood nor could ever actually begin to be fully understood.

Philosophy perhaps is something, or the manner, in a way of speaking, that I contemplate very often.

The technologies, the growths, the advancements of so much that we humans live with and within daily, have changed regularly and frequently the world we live in and the manner as well as behaviors by which we humans live.

It is all fascinating and a process of evolving at a pace and/or rate, which has never before (at least that we know of) been occurring. There is so much good, but there is also so much bad, unfortunately, within. But nature is nature, and we should all recognize such, rather than overlook it and think that everything is clear cut, text book, knowable.

To live one must breathe, to breathe one does not think about it, to think about it can cause hyperventilating. One must be calm and even distract oneself from their own breathing at times. Others must be calm and focus upon their breathing. There is only so much that one can and/or should control, also. With so much that is controllable, there can come a bias and/or misrepresentation, of perhaps what nature is.

When you lose touch with what is being grounded, recognizing that nature is nature and we humans are only one piece within it (it being infinitely larger and of unknown, unknowable proportion/s), then an imbalance occurs. Not only are most all things seemingly inter-related and/or tangled, most all things, regardless, require a balance and according proportion/s.

Discovering

The first time that the words 'Narcolepsy with Cataplexy' appeared
to me was after doing an internet search of the words: "laughter
AND paralysis."

Having been in Mexico for near two weeks, at this point my friend
and I decided to take a quick walk. This was a long-time friend
whom I've known since middle school. At this point in time in
Mexico, I was 28 years old.

We were in Mexico for our good friend's wedding, which was upcoming in a couple of days. The wedding was at the end of the two
week trip, and the wedding couple were staying an extra week
afterward for their honeymoon. The three of us had all grown up in
the same town, all living within blocks of each other. Throughout
high school and college we spent a lot of time together. The friend
who was getting married had traveled with me on many exciting
trips down in Central America, specifically Nicaragua, including the
caravan trip after Hurricane Mitch in 1998. The friend whom I'd
taken this walk with, was sharing/splitting the room with me. We'd
mostly in the past just wandered, riding our bikes some of the time,
around the town. For the first week of the two week trip, the three
of us, along with around a handful of other friends, had traveled
around the Yucatan Peninsula of Mexico, visiting Mayan Ruins.
The trip was excellent, although by this point mid-week two, I was
becoming more than exhausted and was aware that the likelihood
of me collapsing was high.

From around age 20, I'd begun to have odd occurrences where I'd
collapse gradually. Then by age 28, there were many variable
manners in which the odd occurrences were happening. At first,
around 20, they'd only really happen at home when I was either
joking around with, or handing a plate of food I'd cooked over to,

my Mother and Step-Father. The sensation of pleasure from giving them the food I'd just cooked, perhaps surprising them, or just the smiles that they had when I'd hand over the plate was triggering some sort of muscle flickering, weakness, an instant or quickly escalating inability to remain with any strength. At times when I'd say something funny, as soon as my Mother or Step-Father would begin to react laughing, and sometimes it was as I'd myself feel that it was funny, that I'd begin to feel the triggering occurring. Yet, I had no idea for a long while, that there was any triggering of anything going on. During the very first few occurrences, I tried desperately to control it and would just lean over against the door frame in the kitchen, or lean against whatever was nearby, like the arm of the couch. It was odd to me, I had no idea what was occurring, yet it seemed somehow normal to me.

Eventually, after a point, I knew it was not normal. This point was around when I'd stopped being able to remain standing on a few of the occasions. It had kept happening over and over. I'd dropped a few plates of food handing them off to my Mother and Step-Father. Finally, I told my Mother that something odd was happening now and then, which she'd witnessed, that whatever it was, I had no idea why or what was exactly occurring, but that it was entirely beyond my ability to control. She knew exactly what I was referring to, upon my mentioning it. My Mother at first said that she'd thought I was faking it, that she thought I was being dramatic for some reason, trying to draw attention for some/whatever reason. This point in time was probably somewhere around when I was 22 or 23 years old. It had been occurring for a long while at this point. We both knew it was concerning but agreed that it was unlikely there'd be much which could help me or actually rid it, from seeking medical help. She absolutely did not oppose me seeking such; that was my own decision.

It is important for me, at this point, to mention a few things. First off, my medical history is complex and basically from birth has been a roller-coaster. Insurance is something I've had throughout my life, thanks to my Mother who has always insisted upon it and helped me to have it.

Secondly, I've lived with my Mother my entire life. There have only been a few periods when I've lived elsewhere for a few months at a time. She by no means has a lot of money. We really do struggle and juggle month to month, but she is a very hard worker and a very smart person. On the other hand, I am a very strong thinker but have never worked a full time job beyond a few weeks here and there, in my life. This is due to many reasons, not necessarily at all by intent nor because I do not 'want' to. (I want to work; I've tried many roles but none has been manageable and/or tolerable).

Thirdly, from the age of 20 to 28, I did not have a general practitioner doctor. Basically, I'd managed for years to not have anything that wasn't fixable by going to the walk-in clinics and seeing one of the doctors or nurse practitioners there. I'd had a sort of unsatisfying and disconcerting last visit with the general practitioner whom I'd seen up until 20 years old. He basically just didn't want to proceed with analyzing what I'd come in asking him to analyze, although he'd done a brief and basic exam. So, my attitude towards and opinion about seeking medical help was, to put it lightly, not very confident nor re-assuring. And, I chose to not seek such unless something was grave and/or obviously urgent. When I go into my medical history more, perhaps such will help to explain that attitude (?).

So, week two in Mexico, having so much fun and continuing to exhaust myself day after day, again I knew that it wouldn't be long before I collapsed, and I decided to tell both of my good friends the following. It was something along the lines of this: "I want you both to be aware of something odd, please do not be too alarmed and/or worried, if I all cf a sudden collapse. It will likely happen at an odd moment, like when I should be laughing or right as I've maybe said something funny. Know, that I'll be up within a matter of seconds and completely fine. It's been happening for years, but I've managed to not have it happen in public somehow. I'm exhausted and think it may be likely to occur. Just please, don't worry, if it happens." They both were a bit thrown off, but also concerned by what I'd said, yet they knew me well and basically left it at that. However, if I remember right, they both agreed together and told me that I needed to go talk with a Doctor upon returning home. One of them recommended their General Practitioner Doctor to me, and he is who I went to see when I returned home. The friend who I was rooming with in the hotel, was the same friend who recommended his Doctor to me.

A few days into week 2 in Mexico he'd begun to have some stomach matters (this is common and typical when traveling in Central America for any person from the United States, as the water and food can be contaminated). He had been staying in the hotel room for a few days now, dealing with his stomach. Although he'd started to feel better and asked me if I was into walking around, saying he wanted to get out of the hotel for a bit. So, we went for a walk and all was good until on our way back, we were within a block from the hotel and crossing a road when, all of a sudden he just stopped, mid-street. Glancing back at him, since I had stepped beyond where he was, it was very apparent that he was frozen up and extremely awkward looking. At that moment of seeing his face, as quickly as I could, I got to the other side of the street and upon reaching the sidewalk, immediately collapsed. I'd managed to basically collapse against, or onto, a light post as I collapsed to the ground. My friend came rushing over as I collapsed, and was standing above me, very concerned. He was looking right at my face and was very nervous. It was no more than 10-15 seconds before my muscles returned and I was able to lift myself up, laughing as I got up. He wanted to make sure I was okay, and said that it freaked him out, I told him that I was fine and that he should go take care of his business, as I pointed to a restaurant directly next to us. When he went in, I remained sitting down on a bench and thought to myself, okay I've got to figure this out now. It has intruded and is now something that I can not ignore or not manage to explain. While thinking this, I also thought that I should get online at the 'internet cafe' and see what I can figure out, even if it turns out to be meaningless. After my friend came out of the restaurant, I told him that I'd meet him back at the room shortly, after going to the 'internet cafe' to do some searching. He agreed and went on to the hotel.

This was when I did the search, "laughter AND paralysis" and what came back high on the list, was an article about an English lady who when she laughs, goes paralyzed briefly. It was about 'Narcolepsy with Cataplexy' and I was shocked at the similarity of what I was reading, to the odd occurrences which I'd been experiencing for so long. However, 'Narcolepsy' to me seemed crazy, that is to say that I actually believed very much at the time, that I was an excellent sleeper and there was no way that I had some odd 'sleep disorder.' So, with this new set of words, I searched again on the internet and found numerous explanations, as well as definitions, regarding 'Cataplexy.' Finally, I had a word and some understanding to it, although 'Narcolepsy' seemed completely unbelievable, as I'd never fallen asleep mid-sentence...

In ways it was very relieving to have finally had an episode in front of my good friend, and that is the truth. It had been years that I'd had this invisible occurrence, my Mother and Step-Father had witnessed it many many times, but none of my friends had actually seen me collapse. To cause any sort of major concerns towards me, during my friend's wedding week, was definitely not something that I wanted to do but thankfully the friends are wise and level-headed people who took what I said to heart, and did not let it worry them. Maybe it was good, too, that the friend who witnessed it at that point in time, was not the friend actually getting married. Telling them about 'Cataplexy' after reading about it, helped to ease concerns a bit as well, because I described the fact that 'Cataplexy' is quite harmless if the person during the attack/episode does not injure themselves or fall into a position which restricts their breathing, possibly causing real damage. Assuring them that I'd be seeing a doctor promptly upon return was another measure of comfort for them. For myself it was slightly nerving, but I was to a point that I at least needed to discuss things with one and see whether perhaps I was in the ball park, with 'Cataplexy' being the culprit.

For years there had been, so, so many episodes that were subtle and, as I said above, invisible. For instance, a slight droop of the head, a bobbing of the head, a facial spasm, slouching forwards with arms and shoulders, a flinching, a mumble or slurring of my words, leaning against something to brace myself in case of collapse or weakness... These things happened to me almost every single day. They happened during pleasant interactions, during engagements with others, and they also happened a lot while I was skateboarding. When I'd land a trick, or when others would holler or cheer at me after I'd land a trick (a common skateboarder thing to do), such would occur. There were many instances where I had to put my foot down and stop myself abruptly after rolling out of a trick, and then immediately step off of my board and basically just look down at the ground, slouched forwards, for a few seconds. Doing this, or actually laying down as quickly as possible for a few seconds, would dissipate the muscle flickering sensation. My face so often would just droop, somewhat feeling like a facial spasm but actually being facially paralyzed briefly. This I tried to hide because it is not a good feeling, especially when I'm attempting to and needing to smile.

Who knows what people thought, but the fact of the matter is that I didn't care what others thought. Skateboarding is what releases my tensions, it gets the demons out. It is my passion. It has taught me more about nature and life than perhaps any other thing or activity that I've experienced.

Activities which led me into Skateboarding

It wasn't hard to convince my parents to get me a skateboard. Doing so many other activities throughout my childhood, it was just another to add to the list. From a very young age, I'd been playing piano and until around 13 to 15 years old I practiced nearly daily, on many days for hours with my Father. My parents had me doing dance classes, for some reason, before I can even remember, when I was probably between 3 and 5 years old.

Soccer was the first team sport I participated in and played up until around when I got my first skateboard. I played soccer in middle school as well. For a few years in elementary school, I played on a traveling team.

Somewhere between 7 and 9 years old I began Tae-Kwon-Do, and at around 14, I stopped upon completing the black belt test and receiving it.

At somewhere around age 9 or 10, I got a paper route, which I kept until around 16 years old. It was something my parents helped out with often, because getting up so early was never easy for me. On many days I could not do it myself, especially when I had two or three routes for a couple of the years there.

At right around 8 years old, in a large part because of how many others in the small elementary school that I attended were skateboarding, I decided that I wanted to get a skateboard.

It was maybe a year later that I started playing ice hockey, thanks to a skater friend who brought me to an open (ice) skating session. That was one evening after school, and after we'd been skateboarding for hours downtown.

1st Boards & Session/s

Vaguely, I remember being in the large department store and picking out my first board. It was possibly a Nash or Variflex, but more likely just a department store board. It was yellow, flat with a short (actually really none at all) nose. There was a black skull graphic on the bottom; it had both tail and nose guards, with rails as well. My Father was enthusiastic about me learning properly, and he had a good friend whose son Byron (who was around 17 at the time) was a regular skateboarder that knew how to skate well. Arrangements were made for me to meet him and learn the basics. So, we met up at one of the tennis courts on the campus of the university to have a session. The tennis courts had an uplifted section of concrete on one side; it went right up to where the fence was (later I learned this is called a bank, for embankment). Byron was a very friendly and easy to get along with person. I was really excited because he also could obviously skate. First he skated around using the embankment (uplifted section of concrete) and jumping over the sunken tennis net (probably 1' to 2' high at the time). He taught me the basics and I learned to ollie (jump), standing still, just a little on the first day. It was really good and I can remember pieces of that day well. During the session, he had me use his board and he recommended that I get an actual proper and real skateboard, recommending the shop 'Coast Connection' to go to for one.

Soon after the session, I had the money together (from my paper route/s) and went to 'Coast' to buy a proper board. The board I bought was an 'H-Street – Tony Magnusson Mini' Pro-Model with trucks and wheels which I do not remember specifically. Around a year, maybe two, later I got the third board for Christmas, one I'd chosen though, which was a 'Planet Earth – Chris Miller Bird and

Cat' board, one that I wish I could find again as the graphic and shape were so good. There was one more 'old school' board I bought, being another 'Planet Earth – Chris Miller Animal Kingdom' board. Beyond this point, there's been so many I can't begin to remember, and the above mentioned boards were different than the Popsicle shape which has stuck since the early-mid 90's. Byron and I met up one or two other times. At that time Byron was nearing finishing high school and was a musician, a bassist. One day my Father brought me a stack of used boards, which Byron had given him to give to me, since he was moving away to go to school as well as to play bass on a cruise ship that summer. To this day I have the boards he gave me and cherish them because they are thrashed classic boards.

That was the beginning and led to much more. In elementary school there were a handful of other skaters whom I hung out with and some of whom I admired. For years most of those guys kept skating; but as far as I know, today, unfortunately, I am the only one of them all who remains and stuck with it.

Start and Stop, No End

There were a few years, between 8th grade and the end of my freshman year of high school, that I'd stopped skating. Through middle school I'd more or less begun to walk away from playing piano so much, as I'd begun playing the drums for the school band. My Father was supportive, but he never imagined I'd quit the piano (it is his main passion and love in life). Me quitting the piano hurt him, I know; but I have to say my pleasure and interest was skateboarding from here on out. Around my junior year, some friends and I moved a ramp to my yard, a 4' tall mini ramp, 12' wide halfpipe. Soon after this, we moved another ramp, 4' tall with 6' (4' wide) extensions on one end; it was 16' wide in total. We put it a couple of feet from the side of the other mini ramp, creating a gap in-between them. In '95 at 15, during the summer between my sophomore and junior years of high school, a friend and I went to Camp Woodward for one week, where we got to skate new terrain which we'd never before had the chance to skate (a wooden bowl, for instance).

After high school, I got into snowboarding somewhat, and with college I began to be distracted. Plus, some of my skater friends had moved away and many had stopped. So, I stopped again, skating only on some seldom occasions, until three to four years later.

It was about mid-2003, when I heard that our city was finally building a skatepark. At that same time I glanced online and discovered that a skatepark had been constructed, of concrete, in a town around 45 minutes away. Since I had a car and driver's license, a skateboard and energy, it was on. A good friend and I would go to that skatepark at least twice a week, sometimes I'd go by myself a 3rd or even 4th time in a week. Skating again had me stoked, even though I weighed a lot and was quite off (in regards to comfort on the board). It reminded me how much I enjoyed it.

Concrete skateparks are something I'd never experienced and had only seen a few of or dreamed of.

During the construction of our city's skatepark, I went out and introduced myself to the guys building it. Dreamland Skateparks, the main guys responsible for and behind 'Burnside Skatepark' in Portland, Oregon, were who was constructing our skatepark, miraculously. It was an honor to not only meet these guys, but their friendliness and willingness to let me also help out, somewhat, was greatly inspiring. The park was finished up in early '04 (10 years ago almost to this day) and since then, I've not quit skateboarding. There's been a few times that I've had to step back and off for brief periods of time; and I did think that perhaps it was all over, but thankfully it wasn't. Three occasions in particular, first was in '07 when I hurt my knee, second was in '09 after a serious fall which affected my shoulder and neck (it was the worst injury I've had). Then in '11 the Cataplexy had severely interfered and gotten to the point that I did fall once from a complete temporary paralysis (Cataplexy) episode. Thankfully, I've continued to manage still skating, now and then. Definitely I cannot go like I used to; but being able to remain skating, to an extent, helps keep me going. Skateboarding is one of the few things that really help me release the inner-tensions or inner-demons, the stresses and psychological pains which can build up over time.
Playing ice hockey is something that I've come back to doing in the winters for a few years now. I find it can be very therapeutic when all is well (people I'm playing with and proper pace).
Discovering writing has been a very therapeutic form of a similar function, release. Yet, it is totally different.

Skateboarding Basics

To give some insight into the broadness of what skateboarding forces you to learn, I'll go into the basics. When you learn to skate, you take many falls, you must learn to control and balance both the board and yourself. As you gradually learn more and more, the basic things become easier and easier; yet things do not come easy, nor often do they come quickly. The basics are what lead to more and more. You first have to just learn to stand still and control the position of your feet upon the board. Then you need to be able to control the board under your feet, which is to say that you have to hold the board in place with the bottom of your feet and gradually get comfortable with moving your feet around, upon the board. A skateboard will roll back and forth underneath you, if you are not able to stand strong (not stiff); it will shoot out in one direction or the other, and you will fall. That is the most basic thing one must learn, to begin.

After that comes learning to stand on the board while rolling. This is another hard step; but with the first basic task learned, it will be easier than without. For me, having learned to skateboard around the age of 8, it is impossible to even begin to remember exactly and/or imagine that feeling. Perhaps if I were trying to stand up on a surfboard in water, it would be the same sort of unknown difficult task, because I've never been able to try that (unfortunately due to my ears – oh well, I'm thankful to skate). Standing and rolling will require a different sort of balance, compared to just standing still and controlling the board below you. This is where your knees and center of gravity become more at play within the mix. None of what I'm saying, will actually result in someone inexperienced on a skateboard actually being able to just go and do it. Possibly it could help them figure it out, but doing it and practicing it 'hands/feet on' is the only way to learn it.

To throw out just a few more of the basics. There is kicking/pushing to build speed while rolling. Some and most choose to kick with their back foot, while leaving their front foot on the board. This is referred to as 'regular,' as opposed to kicking/pushing with the front foot, referred to as 'mongo.' As you lift your back foot to kick/push, you twist your front foot from being sideways while both feet are on the board, to somewhat pointing your toes towards the front of the board. This is body positioning to allow for strength in the kick, for speed, and is done without thinking, after reaching a point of comfort with enough practice. Using the ball of your foot behind your toes, the twisting of the front foot is simple and easy, eventually very natural.
There is the 'tic-tac,' which is lifting the front wheels up and then down, over and over, as you swing the front end of the board from one side to the other. This is something you do to get comfortable with the board and to get some momentum from a stand still. The point of doing it is to build up rolling, little bit by little bit, not like kicking to get actual speed.
There is carving, which generally is done more commonly on a longboard, or while one is skating skateparks/pools/bowls. Carving is an essential and mandatory basic thing to learn. You use the force of your body weight and positioning to roll, going forwards or turning. The key aspect of it is leaning in one direction, then the other, similarly to a 'tic-tac' but without lifting your front wheels at all.

Like or similar to carving, pumping is the essential function to skating a halfpipe or ramp, any transition or banked obstacle. It is basically pushing down an incline and using gravity along with body positioning, of weight, to build more speed up and/or to maintain whatever momentum you had. It would be easy to go on and on, over the basics of skateboarding.

Tricks begin with an ollie, which is basically jumping from kicking the tail of the deck down with your back toes, or ball of the foot, while jumping simultaneously as you lift your front, with the side of the foot pressing against the grip tape of the board, lifting the board up and off of the ground. On and on...

Falling Basics

There are also techniques that you learn, for falling and/or, of falling. The first element of this is knowing and maintaining awareness of your surroundings, being able to predict (to an extent) which direction and what place will be safe (or safest) to fall towards and upon. For instance, if there is grass on one side of the sidewalk and a gravel lot on the other side of the sidewalk, obviously falling on the grass would be the first choice over the sidewalk, and the gravel lot would be the last choice. Choice is not always an option though when falling; and depending upon whether you hit a rock, or your balance slips, or perhaps you try a trick and do not land it, falling is, simply put, falling.

However, and perhaps this will or will not surprise you, there are methods which can help to 'somewhat' avoid or miss-direct a fall. For instance, there is a method of 'rolling' by putting your front arm out and thrusting your body weight around forwards, so that you actually begin to spin in the fall, thus rolling out of the fall. It is not a common thing to manage though; but the faster you skate and depending upon the tricks that you are trying, as well as the terrain that you are skating, it can and does occur.

Another technique or method, to and/or of falling, is 'running out' and is basically just that. If as you begin to fall you can manage to get the footing along with positioning right, you can end up 'running out' or perhaps, usually awkwardly, stepping out of the fall. It is a quick reflex action but is very common.

When people wear pads, especially knee pads, they learn to go directly to their knees when they fall. This is referred to as the, or a, 'knee slide.' It is commonly used on Vert Ramp skating, when people are skating 8'-12' tall vert ramps (often with 1'-4' + of vertical wall at the peak of the transition). It does save their knees as well as their bodies somewhat, although that is not always possible. Knee sliding ain't easy either. It takes a quick reaction and reflex of basically going to the position of sitting on your knees. There is a lot of difficulty to mastering it due to the vast gravity effects combined with odd contorting that one does while skating. Skaters tend to have a preference and stick to it, of either wearing pads and knee sliding regularly, or of running out of as much as possible without use of any (or with minimal) pads.

You don't see people wearing pads while street skating nor hardly much at skateparks. Why? Because it is uncomfortable and restricting to one's movements, it is often too hot and they become sweaty and gross. Many people don't wear them also because of the fad, or no-pad, mentality. I've worn them plenty in my days but do prefer to not wear them for the reasons of mobility and comfort. It is also hard to 'run out' of things and/or prevent falling altogether, 'running out' of things, that is, when you have a heavy set of pads on your knees. Not to leave out mentioning that knee pads often slide down upon your shins and sometimes don't even keep your knees from becoming scraped up, when you do fall to your knees with them on.

Helmets are a thing of their own. In my opinion there's a time and place for them, depending on the terrain and sessions. Personally, I don't wear one as much as I ought to. At times though, I do wear one. It can be a sensitive subject and, believe me, I've been ridiculed by doctors on such...

Elbow pads can be great. If you've got a tendency to fall on your front hand/s or arm/s, an elbow pad alone can do real wonders. Pads tend to be worn the most, I think, for either Vert skating (as mentioned already) or while healing from a previous injury, to take the impact and/or prevent escalation of something aggravated already.

Tying in Cataplexy

Now, how does Cataplexy tie into all of this? Well, for me I basically gradually adjusted to my Cataplexy with no idea of what nor why it was occurring, over years. It was clear to me soon after it began that there was 'pleasure' involved in its occurring. Now, I know that I should say, rather, pleasure in Cataplexy being triggered.

The sensation of muscles flickering with a sort of aura or sensation in my head was obvious It was only a long while later, after a few real immediate and somewhat intense collapses had occurred, that I realized it was my muscles that were flickering and going more or less paralyzed. The first reaction was to fight it, to remain strong physically resisting and to not let myself fall, and to also continue to laugh and joke around in whatever way I'd been doing forever. But, after a point, I realized that battling it was only causing the Cataplexy to escalate.

There were a few attacks/episodes where I got very frustrated and mad with my body/self. I did all that I could to remain standing and to keep myself from having to stop laughing. These were not good attacks/episodes and were actually the longest and most fierce attacks/episodes, which I've ever had. During one of these I managed to walk from the kitchen, through the living room, and back to my room, where I threw myself onto my bed (more like jumped and had no, 0, muscles by the time that I hit [whip lashing] the bed). When I landed on the bed, it was not good and was actually sort of like a giant belly-flop, with added momentum. Because I'd managed to jump towards the bed, it was with force. In that slight bit of time between jumping and landing, my body had gone entirely limp, and I hit the bed real hard. This made me even more angry and frustrated during the Cataplexy. I mumbled (as I could not speak clearly what so ever) something of rage. My poor

Mother was standing back witnessing this; and as I physically kept fighting/resisting the Cataplexy in the bed for probably 20-30 seconds, my body began to convulse. It was my own doing though, as I was forcing, with any muscle that I could manage to move, to get myself up and to move on (to have my muscles back).
It was after this episode, which only stopped once I got down and let it do its thing (which is to dissipate on its own), that I realized and knew that fighting/resisting the Cataplexy was not a good idea.

Not long after, I decided to try something, which was to try to lay down immediately, as soon as I felt any oncoming of a Cataplexy attack/episode, and to immediately try to focus my thoughts on my body and attempt to relax my body entirely. When the next strong Cataplexy occurred, this plan was in my mind and I tried it. It worked tremendously. The Cataplexy dissipated nearly immediately.

Cataplexy Basics (for me)

These consist of learning to sense the attack/episode oncoming (in the moment, that is). If you can tell that it is going to be an intense attack/episode, getting yourself down onto the ground safely, as quickly as possible may do wonders. Lie down quickly, if you can manage to. Sprawling out and breathing, concentrating on your body is the technique that works for me. It dissipates the attacks/episodes.

Sometimes Cataplexy can hit, leaving me somewhere between frozen and paralyzed. When the freeze occurs, throughout my body I feel odd, as there are sensations of intense flickering. It seems like time slows dramatically and the few seconds that I may remain frozen feel like minutes. In my mind, all that I can do is think, "Am I going to collapse or are my muscles coming back?" During this moment, I am also very much gauging my surroundings and where to fall. It is easy to get frustrated in this frozen state, which doesn't help. Such (any real frustration/s) can only escalate the Cataplexy into an immediate collapse and possibly a hard/er collapse. If you use up whatever minimal strength that remains in the muscles standing still, frozen, and another wave of weakness or the paralysis strikes, you go down like a rag doll. Sometimes though, and it seems like when I manage to breathe while focusing on only my body, my muscles regain strength and I then unfreeze. It is an awfully odd mind and body over the trigger cause, and definitely not something which is consistent (in appearance) or hardly, really describable, depending on the circumstances.

From the many years of having collapsed from Cataplexy and having had my head droop or my body twitch, what I can definitely say is that there is much that one can do to attempt better managing and also minimizing, perhaps, of their own Cataplexy. A lot of that has to do with being aware and conscious of many things and adjusting mannerisms, interactions, as well as behaviors, plus more. That is no simple task. It has a lot to do with lifestyle as well as social engagement/interaction. Some may find this unacceptable and unthinkable, to step away from living life in a common manner. There is definitely no simple path with Cataplexy. It is not possible for me to speak, only, in terms of having just minimal Cataplexy, which may be an occasional head droop. Where I'm coming from, and what I'm speaking about, has a lot to do with collapsing and being briefly paralyzed from head to toe.

Skateboarding with Cataplexy

For years and years, to this day, when I skateboard there are times
and/or occurrences, when Cataplexy hits. There were years during
which it escalated gradually. Years that the Cataplexy was there,
hitting often (daily) while I skated. My head and shoulders would
droop forwards, as soon as I rolled out of a trick, or as others would
holler at me having landed a trick. Somehow, I managed. One
thing was that I did not ignore it, but rather continually as it
occurred, tried to gauge how I could avoid the next occurrence, or
what I could do to minimize it when it happened.
The thing that I sort of figured out was that if I anticipated it
happening, I could basically be ready to engage it -- to step off of
my board and collapse, to use my last bit of muscle strength to stop
my momentum and then fall more safely. There were many times
when this occurred. After rolling out of the trick, I'd start to droop
my upper body and at the moment when I felt like there was still
the strength to manage (which was right away), I'd step down with
my one foot (to stop the momentum, slowing myself down), and
then I'd usually get an arm down to the ground as I sort of semi-
collapsed. There were many occasions where I actually sort of fell,
but it was more of falling to the ground gently, after stopping.
The thing I know and knew then was that if I get down to the
ground safely, then all is good and my muscles will come right
back. If I don't make it to the ground safely, and I actually twist or
impact something on the way down to the ground, then who knows
how bad the Cataplexy may be, or if it may be combined with some
injury(?).
Thankfully, I can still say that I've only had one full out, complete
temporary paralysis episode/attack while on my board. It occurred
when I was very tired skating. I'd not slept well (it was worse than
the usual), and on top of that I'd been doing a lot of interacting that

week and was somewhat stressed as well. What was stressing me out was that I'd been really thinking about the extent of my Cataplexy recently, and how I may actually have to consider basically quitting skateboarding, at age 31. This was such a painful and horrible thing to think about: At 31, that I could no longer do what is my passion in life, and to have not actually hurt myself causing me to have to quit, but rather having to *make a decision* to walk away entirely.

My Cataplexy that year was so intense, I was collapsing repeatedly on many days, anywhere from 5 to 20 times. My poor Mother at home was witnessing many every day. We could not joke around and I had to be very cautious about letting any interactions escalate into either frustration or humor. Never prior had my Cataplexy been so intrusive and/or regular. It was out of control. While at an indoor mini ramp with a skater friend, we were skating very lightly and I'd explained to him where I was at, in terms of how I was frightened by how bad Cataplexy was getting. We'd skated for not very long, maybe 15 minutes and I'd been having a lot of flickers, muscle weakness that would shoot in and out of certain areas of the body, while skating. In a run, I went up and did a basic backside 50-50 grind, both trucks on the coping, grinding with my back to the deck of the ramp. When I locked into the grind, the Cataplexy hit, and hard. Basically, I was immediately completely paralyzed. Luckily as this happened, my momentum and angles were just right, in that as I went falling, I went straight downwards and my body managed to slide right into, then down the transition. Had I fallen straight downwards like that, say 2 or 3 inches behind where I was, more towards the deck, I would have smacked the steel coping very, very hard with some part or parts of my body. Such would not have been good. After the fall, at the bottom of the transition, I remained down for a few seconds as the Cataplexy dissipated. My friend was staring at me oddly. Immediately upon my muscles returning, I grabbed my board and stepped off of the ramp, telling my friend "that's it, I'm done, it's happened."

From that point on I went for a few months, not skating even once. It was another 6 months or so after that, before I began skating somewhat regularly again, this was in a large part from having begun certain lifestyle adjustments. Over those first few months I thought hard and deep on everything. The thought of only being 30 and having to quit skateboarding entirely, my passion, was devastating. I'd already walked away from so much, I'd recognized what was occurring for years and had adjusted to it all, as best that I could. In my mind, I'd expected to be skating perhaps even to some minimal extent into my 50's and possibly even beyond. The idea of letting back, slowing and/or minimizing the intensity, of course was something I knew would be coming up before long. Although, I have a few friends who are in their 40's and they are still going quite strong, even progressing and becoming better at skateboarding. Those few months off were rough, they were strange and somewhat unfamiliar. Not only was the impact of not skateboarding causing things to be odd, but the extent of the Cataplexy being as bad as it had gotten, was having effects throughout all aspects of my living.

This was when I had to walk away from my top career choice which I'd been getting heavily into, building concrete skateparks.

A friend in Denmark that I'd helped with design numbers for the bowl they were preparing to construct, offered me a paid flight plus all accommodations and even money to come work constructing the bowl. Because of the frequency and the extent of my Cataplexy, collapsing multiple times each week if not each day, I sadly was as upfront as possible in turning down the offer due to the Cataplexy.

It was a big bummer for me, and my friends involved were also bummed. It would have been too risky though, and I know that I would have been a risky burden. Passing up the first and only opportunity I've had to go to Europe was and remains, super painful.

In the end though, I did help a little bit and did connect my Danish friend with my good local skater/builder friend, who flew out and led the construction of the bowl which is now complete!

Today, experiencing so much less Cataplexy, I'd jump aboard and give it my best. Recently, I've been involved in some skateparks conceptual design work, working with my good friend who has started Hunger Skateparks. It is really good to be involved to the extent that I can manage.

Cataplexy – Idiopathic Central Sleep Apnea – Escalation

It was a few months later (after the skateboarding fall from Cataplexy) that, thankfully, I could note that my Cataplexy had begun to slightly lessen.

There is much more to the story of what was going on with the Cataplexy having escalated so badly, such related directly with having been using a 'sleep-breathing device/machine' to attempt helping my minimal-moderate 'Idiopathic Central Sleep Apnea.' Such took place over 9 months, the worst 9 months of my life. It took a few months of being off of the machine for the Cataplexy to regress, more or less, back to what it had been prior to beginning that 9 months.

It took traveling to Mayo Clinic in Rochester, MN, before being able to get off of the breathing machine at night, which seemed to be at the root of my Cataplexy having become so bad. For three weeks, I stayed in a hotel with a small kitchenette, basically across the street from a Target store where I grocery shopped. I'd taken a train to Rochester, MN, because I was worried about driving that distance, along with having had a sort of discouraging interaction with the neurologist's 'physician's assistant, who'd been overseeing me (neglecting to hear me in regards to the Cataplexy escalation and ENT effects also occurring) over the 9 month time frame. Being in that hotel and going to Mayo Clinic as much as I did was an experience, in and of itself; not one that I'd like to have to go through again.

In the end though, after the three weeks, after being analyzed and seen by neurologists, the sleep specialists and briefly by an ENT, the breathing machine was said 'to not be benefiting me' and I was able to discontinue use of it.

Within months of being off of the machine, my Cataplexy began to subside. Still, it took another year and many, many lifestyle adjustments, which I made gradually, before getting to more or less where I'm at now, which is a much better place in regards to Cataplexy and all things.

Today, I occasionally will sleep using my Pulse Oxymeter. It is an overnight one, which I can plug into my computer to check how my sleep was, in regards to both my blood oxygen saturation levels and also my pulse rate. Being that I have Idiopathic Central Sleep Apnea, one huge adjustment I made to help limit the amount of apneas was having (or will have), was learning to sleep on my side rather than on my back. When one sleeps on their back, they are much more likely to have apneas while asleep. An apnea involves not breathing, or stopping breathing, for over 10 seconds. There are multiple reasons which relate to both the tongue obstructing, and/or the throat airways constricting. Know that, by sleeping on your side, you are much less likely to have apneas. Also know that, everyone now and then will have apneas, it is not entirely avoidable, when one is congested they tend to have more of them. Sleep Apnea can be very problematic, especially over time as it can keep one from achieving proper, or healthy, sleep; breaking the sleep cycle in a different manner, but similar manner, like Narcolepsy. Many people benefit greatly from using the breathing machines/devices (CPAP, BiPAP, VPAP). Always be aware of what you're getting into though.   Remember that if you seem to have what is called a 'minimal' (less than 10-15 apneas hourly) sleep apnea matter after a Polysomnography (sleep study), prior to trying a machine/device take some basic steps and simple adjustments to improve your sleep quality. Specifically learn to sleep on your side and not your back, you can place a pillow behind your back, or even tie it with a string around your belly and/or chest...

Lifestyle Adjustments

Over time these, more or less, are the lifestyle adjustments that have appeared to work the best for me. At least, that is, so far.

Day to day, I must do my best to stay on the path. Such can be difficult and requires continual observation, along with frequent maneuvering. And, there are pot-holes, struggles, barriers, here and/or there.

There will always be the unknowns which exist, as there will always be potential for interferences and/or obstructions on any path. One must remain strong, focused and in-tune with themselves. Continually weighing as to what is affecting them, be it positively and/or negatively, and focusing in on what or in which manner/s are those effects.

Juggling is crucial and not always so easy, but in time and especially with devoted practice (focusing), one does learn.

Persons who have Narcolepsy with Cataplexy spend a lot of time adjusting. Very often this occurs while they are nearly completely blind to 'it' going on (be 'it' whatever pertinent circumstance/s that relate to the adjusting, or be 'it' having Narcolepsy).

Subconsciously that (adjusting) is not only exhausting but can be another large element of what goes on deep within. These initial adjustments are an element which really drains the person, in ways, of both their mental and physical strength/s.

Many of the disease symptoms can be so obscure and/or are tied so deeply, into so much that is common and normal in everyday living of life, that one who has Narcolepsy can and/or does eventually place the symptom/s and their effect/s on the back burner of their focus. Eventually the person is not necessarily in any way focusing on the symptom/s or the symptom/s effect/s, but rather the person is basically putting all of their focus and strength/s elsewhere. That elsewhere typically has to do with just getting through life in some so-called 'normal' manner.

Perhaps what the person who has Narcolepsy thinks is 'normal' functioning, based on their own functional abilities and life experience, is, in fact, often very much not normal functioning in regards to the general society. The persons functioning level/s can be entirely out of the ordinary, comparably speaking. This applies, too, to their thought of what it means to function "normally" with respect to others.

The most common and upfront, yet difficult, example of this would be relating to what would be considered 'normal tiredness.' When 'being tired' can mean exhausted, sleepy, lethargic and much more, it becomes hard to interpret and/or use the word 'tired' universally speaking. However, the obvious is for 'tired' to mean that the person feels a need to rest.

Once the person knows that they have Narcolepsy and has an understanding of what it actually is, much recognition as well as realization/s can quickly hit.

How a person with Narcolepsy regularly feels is often described by the medical experts as being equivalent to how a person without Narcolepsy feels after not having slept for 48 - 72 hours. When you live for years, nearly daily having such a cloud of sleepiness sometimes on and off, coming and going throughout the day, day to day, you become accustomed to it, in whatever vast ways (positive and/or negative).

It is very important that one who has Narcolepsy, especially, be able to stay connected with their own reality and not become disconnected from it. To block out the subconscious and to ignore your gut (too often) is a mistake. That may sound a bit wacky, but it has to do directly with how stresses and anxieties play into so much in life, as well as having to do directly with how much the person plays into, or reacts to, those stresses and anxieties.

Remember that any and all stresses, pressures and anxieties upon persons with Narcolepsy tend to have heavy and obscurely complex consequences.

To add a bit more, which I know may be going far off, I'll add the following. So many of the typical societal procedures, standards and processes are very complex. But most are nearly always portrayed, considered and/or played upon as being 'normal.' This includes things to do with so, so much that goes on in our daily living of life, be it career-oriented, social inter-activity, interpersonal communications, finances, etc..., much of which are crucial to one's well-being and/or general stability and things that directly often produce stress. Falling into this are money, education, health, career/s, relationship/s, shelter, etc...

Caution is mandatory and care is essential to managing stress and to ever finding a general stability.

For myself today, I have no desire (0) to run any race/s.

Running endless races was how I grew up, as it seemed to be a never ending race, right up until around the end of college. It was all I knew. Did I realize that I was really, really tired, or that I was *racing? No. However, I sure noted the fatigue, most all of the time. What else did I note? All too frequent headaches and major difficulties with completing so many things that I felt were necessary to do, that is, the things which I thought would bring me general stability in the long term: having a full time job and eventually finding my career, moving away from my home (out of my Mother's home), meeting a partner and having a relationship (perhaps one day having children and a family), eagerly participating in community activities or events (at least now and then), helping parents as they age, traveling as much as possible, etc... Those were a few of my dreams and/or aspirations at that time.*

Of the above, I basically have chosen slivers of them to be happy with. Perhaps one day I can pursue them further and/or have them fall into place, if it happens naturally. But, I do not have the drive to run, race nor fight for much any of it. That was something I had to finally accept and was not for me necessarily a tough thing to accept.

Narcolepsy with Cataplexy is what it is, and will be what it will be. All that I can do is make the most of what I can. What I do is what I can manage, and what I don't do is what I cannot. Sure, there are limitations to what I can do; but there are, simply put, also limitations to that which can be done.

Time and space are really still very much unknowns, like sleep. To my mind, life has as much to do with the reflections that go on everywhere as it has to do with the connections which occur all of the time.

Having general stability requires the proper proportioning of what is or may be necessary, along with the proper balancing of what is required.

The following is something I wrote thinking on Skateboarding, but pertaining to much, much more...

Nothing has taught me more, nor allowed me to explore.
Practice is required for whatever is desired.
Often what is desired may not be of what is required.
What is required depends on more than that which is desired.
Reaction can be acquired, although only with the desire.
Instinct is of importance when reaction is important.
Advancement, takes complacence, along with patience.
Relaxed and calm, patience is strong.
Strong is, not thinking, and is, simply being.
Strong thinking, can distort, also contort.
Awareness is key, as balance needs to be free.
Proportion is no distortion and requires proper contortion.
Contortion is absorption, yet without inappropriate distortion.
Inappropriate distortion can result in improper contortion.
Absorption is natural and of instinctive reflex reaction.
Knowing is not necessarily growing.
Going, as well as growing, takes rolling.
Rolling is the first step to knowing, on one's way to growing.
Proportion is relevant in every element.
For every element, one must focus on the crucial relevance.
Dissecting relevance takes observing relation and continual contemplation.
Connecting relevance is thought, from dot to dot, and not, knot to knot.
With conscious calm and relaxed thought, you always roll; onwards, and on words.

Acupuncture / Cupping / Osteopath

A friend of mine had many times suggested that I visit his osteopath, a Korean doctor well practiced in both ancient Eastern medicines as well as modern Western medicines. His specialty is acupuncture and blood-letting cupping. His Father practiced Eastern medicine in Korea for many years and had taught him from a young age. The osteopath had taken part in many books, diving into Eastern medicine, specifically blood-letting cupping. The friend of mine, along with his Father, had been seeing this osteopath for many years. They live near him and are friends of his, as well as patients who drive an hour to see him at his office.

It sort of happened unexpectedly that I went along with my friend to one of his appointments. My friend's wife has Fibromyalgia and other quite persistent, somewhat at times serious, health matters. She highly recommended that I set up an appointment.
Then out of nowhere one day, my friend called me and said he was in town. He'd been living to the north around 12 hours away for a few years and I'd not seen nor talked with him hardly, since he'd moved. When he called, he invited me to have lunch with him and his wife. I accepted and met up with them promptly. At the lunch I discussed a lot of what I'd been going through, the discovering of Narcolepsy with Cataplexy, along with how much it sort of helps explain many of my mannerisms and even my character, in so many ways. They discussed many of the matters they'd been going through as well, including the Fibromyalgia, along with how difficult certain times are. Where they're living is very desolate and far away from any large hospital or city with diversification as far as doctors goes. It's been difficult for them to find a doctor. The osteopath came up in the conversation, and they told me that they were actually going to see him after lunch. His office is in the state

capital, a one hour drive to the north. My friend offered to let me come along to meet the osteopath as well as to see what he does, because blood-letting cupping was something odd and something I was entirely unfamiliar with. Since I had a real interest and nothing else going on, I accepted the invitation.

At the office of the osteopath, in the patient room with my friend, immediately once the doctor had come into the room, it was very apparent that they were good friends. The doctor was asking him about his new life and house, where he had moved to. Watching the blood-letting cupping was quite an experience though. After acupuncture is done and you are still on your back (typically), a needle-pen-like tool is first used to puncture small holes in the skin where the cup is later placed. A small rolled up piece of paper is lit on fire with a lighter and then put within the glass cup, which is placed solidly on the body, where the skin has been punctured. The glass cups come in a variety of shapes and sizes. The cups remain on the skin for 10 minutes, as you lay on the stomach. During the first minute especially, blood seeps out into the cup, then it mostly settles and the pressure remains on the skin. After the 10 minutes expire, the nurse comes in and removes the cups. Carefully she uses clothes to wipe off and clean the blood before she rubs a cream on the locations. The appearance of the skin where the cups were placed is odd. There are purple and/or red circles, bruises, which remain for days. There is significance to the color of the circles, as well as the blood that is removed; it relates to the toxicity of what was removed from the body as well as to the extent or quality of one's blood circulation.
Anyways, I was both a bit surprised by what I'd seen as well as intrigued and interested in attempting such. So, as I left that day with my friend and his wife, I set up an appointment.

The appointment was for one week later and it was definitely worthwhile. This osteopath did a lot more for me than just the acupuncture and blood-letting cupping, thankfully.

He immediately recommended that I attempt to cleanse for a few months, by going gluten free as well as dairy free, along with no sweets; and he told me to walk at least one mile each day, and also to be sure to drink plenty of water daily.

So, after the first cupping experience, I began changing up my diet. Each two weeks I went and received acupuncture and blood-letting cupping.   I did such for around 5 to 6 months.

Within 3 months of my first visit with the osteopath, I'd lost around 15-20 pounds.   I'd fallen under 200 pounds for the first time in over 10 years. Beyond that, I was feeling very good. My Cataplexy had regressed by the end of those 3 months to the point that it had been, more or less, prior to starting the breathing machines which caused me so much havoc. At this point I'd become quite impressed and was more open to some of what the osteopath was recommending. The osteopath gave me some Chinese medicine to take. They were alternative forms of the medicine used for Cataplexy, antidepressants. Being quite reluctant, but at this point convinced that perhaps this would be worthwhile, I attempted such. Really, the fact that what he was giving me were natural plant substances versus something more unknown or simple, to me brought a bit more confidence in attempting the treatment.

It was a 3 month course of two types of medicines that he recommended and I took. The ingredients in one of the meds were 5-HTP, Taurine and L-Theanine. The medicines did give me bits of energy. I was able to skateboard with more strength and definitely was feeling good, in that Cataplexy was not interfering with me skating. But, there was another side to it. I was noticing that out and about, Cataplexy was being triggered quicker and maybe stronger. When I was asked questions about directions on the street one day, Cataplexy struck quite hard, freezing me up. Here's another example. There were a few homeless guys who always ask me for change, and typically the Cataplexy I experience during these interactions is of a minimal head droop or sort of rumble in my knees. But the usual head droop had become more of a freeze and/or collapse.

So, things had flipped a bit. I was stronger during physical activity but more vulnerable during interactions. Because of this oddness, I do not plan on taking the medicines again. But I am glad that I did attempt them; and who knows, perhaps someday down the road, if things get real bad, I may be open to them again.

As for acupuncture and blood-letting cupping, I think they were good for me at the time. Every few months, or maybe even just once a year, I intend to have them done. Acupuncture and/or massage, I think, are great therapeutically. If they were more affordable, I would definitely try to have one or both weekly. There are physical and mental benefits from both. I've definitely felt better for a while after having either done.

Allergies – Seasonal / Perennial

Having had so many headaches and migraines so often throughout my childhood, it seemed as though I'd never get over them. When I was young they were super intense, sometimes with vomiting, deep throbbing, like being stabbed in the temple. As I got older the aches lowered into my neck and shoulders as well, often feeling as though my neck needed to snap in some position to be corrected. Yet the pain would go in waves up into my head and then back down to my shoulders.

Through elementary school especially, I took acetaminophen and ibuprofen multiple times a week, and often multiple times on whichever day/s. By the end of high school I'd found they'd not helped, so I weaned off of them gradually. However, I should mention that I had some serious dental work done in my junior year, which resulted in being given stronger medicines containing acetaminophen (Vicodin).

Not only did I have the more typical dental matters like wisdom teeth removals and cavity/filling work done, but also my upper front left tooth was knocked out while playing one-on-one basketball, fooling around in the gym at school one day with a good friend. It's a bit comical to look back on with my friend, but it was a real ordeal. Having a dentist use a rubber mallet the size of a baby's fist, to get the metal implant up and into the upper jaw bone properly is itself a painful memory.

Basically, from thereon for years, I kept my pain medicines from dental matters for when I had my more serious headaches and would only take them otherwise, minimally, when really necessary for dental or other pains. Eventually though, such medications stopped working. They might temporarily rid the headache, but then it would actually come back much more fiercely later that day or the next day.

The thing that has always helped my headaches is ice. Today ice and rest, or attempting to rest, is what I do when I get a bad headache. As I went through my 20's the headaches had become less intense but more frequent. They were at times almost constant and went on for days on end, a dull ache, sometimes pulsating and other times throbbing, coming and going out of nowhere. At 30, I was still dealing with them too frequently. At the time, I had become so much more in focus regarding the overall picture of my health, due to the discovery of more than likely having Narcolepsy with Cataplexy (as Cataplexy was very apparent, though the other Narcolepsy symptoms were still not yet).

When I was 30, I underwent ENT allergy testing and I reacted to the following:
Seasonal – Trees: Tree Mix A (Ash, Walnut, Sycamore), Tree Mix C (Cottonwood, Elm, Maple), Black Willow, Birch, Oak. - Grasses: Johnson, K.Y. Bluegrass, Bermuda. - Weeds: Ragweed, English Plantain, Weed Mix (Yellow Dock, Burweed, Rough Marshelder, Cocklebur, Lambs Quarter, Sheep Sorrel), Grain Pollen (Wheat, Corn, Barley). - Dust: Grain Mill Dust.
Perennial (Year-Round) – Dust: House Dust, Dust Mites F., Dust mites P., Cockroach Mix [no reaction to Paper Dust and Cotton Linters]. - Molds: Alternaria, Hormodendrum, Cephalsporium, Penicillium, Helminthosporium [no reaction to Pullularia, Aspergillus and Fusarium]. - Fungals: Candida, Epidermophyton, Trichophyton. Animal Danders: Cat [no reaction, amazingly, to Dog, Horse and Feathers (Chicken, Duck, Goose)].

So, in summary, of the 34 things on the list, I reacted to 29 of them. This was kind of shocking to me, being that I'd never let such seem to be an influence on anything; yet, I knew very well from my childhood that my brother suffered seriously from, seasonal allergies, at least. My brother moved away from home right out of high school and within a handful of years' time, had moved out to California where he loves living, in part because he doesn't suffer from the allergies like he had here. As a child I remember my Mother and brother both getting regular allergy shots, this was while I was frequently dealing with ear infections and tubes.

The ENT allergy technician talked to me about allergy shots, which I was and still am not interested in. She also described how I should attempt to eat accordingly with the seasons and also to monitor pollen counts online to gauge whether or not I should go out and do whatever activity outdoors. She described how she uses a lot of Benadryl, frequently, and also irrigates her nasal cavities with a Neti-Pot a couple of times daily. Such was all to help her keep her allergies mostly controlled.

She also told me that getting rid of my cats might help, to which I instantly smirked and said, "No way."

From this realization though, of being allergic to so much, I began a long and gradual striving to limit and avoid allergens. First, I decided that from then on I would keep the two cats out of my bedroom (which is where my computer is and also where I spend most of my time).

Second, I read up on ways to minimize and eliminate allergies. A few of the recommendations which I still follow are using hypoallergenic mattress and pillow covers, not hanging clothes outdoors to dry (which I'd always done), removing clothes and rinsing hair after being outdoors, etc. Thirdly, I decided I'd test the waters of certain things to try to get a grasp on what triggers what. Around this time I'd been enjoying hiking, as much as I could manage. So what I did was after a couple of different hikes in the

woods (mid-summer) upon returning home, I gauged some things, like what happened if I did nothing, versus changing clothes after a quick shower along with a nasal irrigation. How would I feel two hours later (?).
Within days it was very clear to me how sensitive I really was/am to the seasonal Allergies. Thankfully, I was able to tell a real difference in feeling quite a bit better and/or recovering much quicker, when I did change my clothes after showering and irrigating my nose.

Something I think is very important to mention, in regards to nasal irrigation, is that you have to be very careful, specifically, about what water you use (there are real dangers when using just straight tap water), and always to be sure to clean the Neti-Pot thoroughly prior to every use.
What I do is use water that has been filtered through the Berkey Filter which we have. I put about a cup into the water boiler and warm it. As that warms I fill the Neti-Pot with about half a cup of water, 1/8 tsp of finely ground Himalayan salt (it is the only salt I consume, unless out and about) and add a pinch of baking soda. Lastly I add the warm water and shake to mix well.
There are three techniques that can be used with a Neti-Pot. They are not easy to explain, but I'll try to minimally do so here. Each of the techniques works in a different manner, affecting/cleansing different areas of the nasal cavities. The first and easiest method is to turn your head sideways and simply pour into the higher nostril (with head turned) and let the water-mix make its way out the lower nostril; then turn your head the other way and do the same. The second method isn't hard compared to the third, but is a bit harder than the first method. You press one nostril closed and insert the Neti-Pot (with head and Neti-Pot tilted enough that the

water-mix is ready to flow in) and then inhale gradually through the nostril with the Neti-Pot within. This is a very odd sensation, as the water-mix travels up through the nasal cavities which go up into one's forehead. The water-mix makes its way down and into your mouth. The third and last method is difficult. I actually can't hardly do it. Basically it is the second method, but in reverse. You pour the water-mix into your mouth and breath it in and up your nasal cavities, forcing it up and out of your nostrils. Be very careful with any of these.

In my opinion, personally, I do not like to irrigate my nose more than a few times a month. Yet when allergies are real bad I do it sometimes a couple of, or a few times, in a week here and there. Another thing that I was told by an ENT Doctor at Mayo Clinic, who checked my ears, nose and throat, was to inhale Sesame Oil, to prevent dryness (for instance, during the winter) and to help the nasal cavities heal. (A year prior to seeing this ENT, I'd had a Septoplasty with Turbinate Reduction and Myringetomy Tubes put in. He could still see areas in the nose healing and suggested such).

Another Doctor told me that mineral oil could be used in helping to clean the ears of ear wax, yet this is something I've not done.

Food Allergies / Sensitivities

To get back into allergies, food is unfortunately a large piece of it. At 31, it had been around six months from when I first saw the doctor of osteopathy who recommended that I try going gluten free and dairy free. This was a year out from having been collapsing 5-20 times daily from Cataplexy; and having been through such a wringer trying to find benefits from treatments, I was now though, on my way upwards. I'd been collapsing less and less from Cataplexy, yet I was still collapsing at times and experiencing regular minimal Cataplexy. Regardless, I was motivated and I found most everything the osteopath was doing to be beneficial (apart from the meds I'd tried). So, I decided I would give it my all to try, for at least a few more months, being gluten and dairy free.

Cooking has always been something that I did not find too annoying and/or tedious. Sure, there are times where there's nothing I'd rather not do, but I've always sort of found it to be no big deal. If there's nothing pressuring or distracting me from the tasks involved, I have no problem cooking. My diet had always involved a lot of meat, and I decided it was time to try to change this up, to an extent. At first, it was difficult to not want meat in every meal but, before too long I adjusted and was fine with eating meat just two or maybe three times a week (rather than as the main part of nearly every meal, multiple times a day). Shitake mushrooms in place of meat in the meals I cooked, really helped me get over the high meat consumption (addiction). Bread has not been something I eat too regularly. However it is something one misses when they cannot indulge it with ease. Thankfully, there are legit gluten free alternatives when it comes to flours and breads and/or pastries, whatever. There are great brown rice noodles out there. Cheese though, on the other hand, oh man, is so so good and there are absolutely no cheese alternatives that come anywhere near matching the real thing. Milk has always been something I've drunk pretty regularly, so eliminating it was a bit tough. Yet thankfully there are many alternatives which definitely do the trick (almond, soy, rice milks, for example). Eating according to the season is something I try to do, yet I still cook pretty much whatever feels right at the time I'm deciding to cook. To the extent that I can manage, I do garden; and I also often attend the Farmer's Market and keep an eye on what is fresh or current (so to speak, to the season). Cooking nearly everything that I eat takes typically an hour to two daily, which is fine at this time for myself. I cook for my Mother and myself. Very often I cook meals large enough to have 1 day, or maybe 2 days-worth of leftovers from. Snacks are needed frequently; and it doesn't take long, maybe 15 or 20 minutes, to come up with something quick.

What I eat regularly as snacks: guacamole, hummus, chips (corn), apples with honey and cinnamon, banana, pineapple, watermelon, celery with nut butter, nuts or trail mixes, dried mango or apricots (non-sulfured), kale, peas, cereals, dark chocolate [85%+]...
One of the biggest things that I realized triggers my headaches and/or migraines are sugars. Unfortunately, the sugars seem to be the types in almost any processed food and/or candy. Almost any store bought juices, especially orange juices, will give me a near immediate headache. The same goes for coffee, I've never been able to drink Folgers, gas station or fast food, coffees.
One definite instance is if I get a Starbucks coffee and add either any of their syrups (chocolate, for example) or even a drop of their soy milk (which is not Silk, it is their own manufactured soy milk), within seconds of taking a sip, a headache hits. Usually these are very dull waves of aching, coming up from my shoulders, around

the top of my head and straight to the back of my eyes, throbbing and/or stabbing. My eyeballs can feel like they're growing and shrinking. Such can be there for hours from just a small sip. Unfortunately, I'm unable to consume so much as I once did, because of this allergy to what specifically I don't even know (¿sugar cane, MSG salt, the processing facility, contaminants?). It's okay though. Not being able to buy junk food only saves me from spending money that I don't have to begin with!

Things I've found that are fine and delicious are fresh or frozen fruits (natural only), high end – dark chocolate (85%+), and raw honey. In the summer when it is hot, I blend ice with frozen fruits and a bit of water for an ice cold smoothie. Another good thing in the summer is making popsicles.

Food, Shopping, Balancing & Cooking

In the day and age we're living in, there is so much danger that exists within what is in front of each and every one of us, be it blatant and/or disguised.

I am not going to try to get into any conspiracy stuff, but I will describe what I feel is important to at the least consider and/or be aware of. There have been over the last 10 years many comparisons of today's food industry to yesteryear's (and today's still) tobacco industry. Begin thinking on it by taking a couple of crucial examples. Take what is essential, with the main ingredients in almost all common foods being both salts and sugars. Think of both monosodium glutemate (MSG) and high fructose corn syrup. Maybe, likely, you are familiar with the scandals relating to both and the negative health effects of consuming high amounts of either and/or especially both, over time.

Unfortunately, they are in so many foods still being processed today. Maybe, more than ever? Why? Because there's been vast manipulation of what labeling is necessary as well as of what words represent what. Just yesterday I read something about how nearly every single large pizza company continues to use large amounts of MSG in their core ingredients of the dough. The companies have put serious efforts into keeping that fact from being known.

Again, I am not trying to get too deep here in any conspiracy direction. But when you see something labeled 'beef patty' you must consider that it may not actually have any real beef in it, or perhaps that, yes, it may include some beef, but how much, and of what, or which part/s (?).

So, I try to avoid regretting what I eat, not only because of what headache I may get, but because some of the ingredients used so commonly are downright dangerous in large quantities and over time. (Take gluten, for example, which, in brief, is a protein taken from wheat and used to fatten foods, be that why it is so essential for bread.)

Today, I don't get near the headaches that I was getting most all of my life prior to the diet changes. Definitely, I am thankful and attempt to remain thankful. How do I do such? Well, it ain't easy, and unfortunately today the cheaper options are most always (80%+ of the time) the unhealthier options. Also, cooking nearly everything that I eat myself is huge in how I manage.

Considering what I need to avoid (sugars, gluten, dairy), I buy food accordingly. Because I don't cook prepared (processed) meals, I buy ingredients individually and with close examination, using caution to avoid what I know will be problematic. Usually I walk out of the store with straight vegetables and fruits. Often I have gluten free corn chips, too. I am not going to get into Genetically Modified Organisms (GMO's) here, but I will say that I attempt to avoid them as much as possible.

Organic fruits and vegetables will be better than the non-organic, in my opinion. Yet, I do buy non-organic specific items often (for example, avocados, tomatoes, etc.). Picking and choosing can be a juggling act and prices do play into it, as well.

When it comes to organic, I feel strongly it is more important when it comes to eggs and meat. I do not want to eat meat that is not locally grown and organic, without antibiotics or growth hormones. The amount of contaminants in today's common meats and foods is scary. If you don't believe it, please do a little research into metals in meats, or how Methicillin-Resistant Staphylococcus Aureus (MRSA) seems to have developed (only) in the pig farms that were injecting high amounts of antibiotics and growth hormones into the pigs. There's much factual information out there about it all.

Unfortunately, when there's a profit to be made, there can be power; and care, along with general safety, can be flung out the window, or laid to rest...

When I cook, I use a lot of spices and herbs of all types, especially Indian and Latin spices. Specifically, for vitamin/supplemental/health reasons, I like to consume a lot of turmeric (I add to stir fry, soups, etc.) and cinnamon (I add a fair amount to my coffee daily). Another thing I've done is gone to decaf coffee, which was due to over-active bladder matters and sometimes headaches were clearly relating to caffeine.
Almost all the oil that I use is unrefined coconut oil.
Within a few months of beginning the gluten and dairy-free changes, I'd lost 20-30 pounds and Cataplexy had lessened even more, not to mention that I was clearly noting much less of the general fatigue that I'd been regularly feeling for years, since high school.
There were many more benefits that gradually became clear. Such as, my general mood and/or attitude had improved. For years, if not as far back as high school or earlier, I could easily snap and become very rude or just over-dramatic towards my Mother. Usually, this would be in response to something petty or even nothing at all, just me having a sort of moment (many of them over the years). Many times, during these moments that I'd have of frustration, I would be at the same time just sort of knowing or thinking of how silly I was being. For years, I'd easily noted my own doing such, being rude and/or just silly stubborn over really nothing. For instance, deciding on what to eat when I was really hungry, would sometimes turn into this long-dragged-out ordeal of whining about it, rather than simply going into the kitchen and preparing something/anything.

It really was a big step to have made it through getting beyond such, and it is one that I definitely look out for occurring again, as I feel totally silly when I reach such a point anymore. Over time snacks became straight kale (!mmm!), guacamole with (gluten free) chips, perhaps an apple or some pineapple.

It all comes down to proportion and balance. Finding each is complicated and, of course, they are also always fluctuating. My food palate has grown so much over the past few years. Today I eat many, many more varieties of food than before. Foods that I'd not have eaten with ease a few years ago, or even more recently (as my palate continues to grow), include brussel sprouts, squash, eggplant, zucchini, kale, bok choy, kiwi, salmon, avocado, and much more. All YumMm..!

Sleep Hygiene
Sleep hygiene is hugely important for someone who has
Narcolepsy. It consist of the following factors: being/having
comfort, having silence (or masking external noise/s – using a fan,
white noise, soft music, etc.), having darkness, having a proper
temperature which you comfortably can sleep within, naps, and
importantly following a semi-strict sleep schedule and routine.

Forever I've been a late nighter and late morning sleeper. Falling
asleep before midnight has hardly ever been easy for me. Mayo
Clinic diagnosed me with Delayed Sleep Onset (or Phase) Disorder
which is a circadian rhythm sleep disorder. People with it fall
asleep late and wake up late, compared to the general population.
It affects the timing of sleep, core body temperature rhythm, and
alertness peak periods. At this point in time, I don't consider it to be
problematic, since I'm not pressured with any schedule and can get
the sleep I need, as it is needed. However, I do try hard to stick to a
general sleep schedule and routine. What I try to do is just be in
bed within the same few hours each night, and to not wake up too
late in the day. When I can manage to, I do like to get some
morning (gentle) sun.
One thing that I've not done for years is try to force myself to fall
asleep or to very often get into bed when I am not tired (unless I'm
dealing with a headache). What years ago developed, as far as
going to bed, is that when I feel the tiredness is there, or when I
begin nodding off (if it begins to happen out of nowhere), I shut
down or turn off whatever and step into the bathroom to quickly
brush my teeth. Then I step over into my bed (both being no more
or than four steps from my desk).
When I feel heavy sleepiness hitting or oncoming, usually this is at
least a few days each week, I take whatever nap that is necessary.

Usually they're not more than 2 or 3 hours and not often do I need two in a day, yet there definitely are those days. As far as when I need the random nap, is complete randomness, sometimes within the first couple hours of awakening and other times it's in the evening, or in between. Sometimes, I can manage to focus my attention enough so onto something, of interest, that I can avoid having to take a nap; as I know it is not good to sleep too much, but often it is pretty much a necessity.

My bedroom has two large windows and a door with a large window, but it remains fairly dark in the mornings, which is a good thing for me. Unfortunately, I cannot damper the sound of the street in front of the house though, and living two to three blocks away from the hospital definitely has its sirens' annoyance factor. There's not a lot I can do about the noise. I've looked into ear plugs, but with the sensitivities or vulnerabilities that I have for ear infections, I don't like to take the chance with them. Sometimes I'll turn on the air filter in my room, which has a fan, to make a background noise (usually I'll turn it on when my tinnitus is at an annoying pitch) for when I'm going to sleep. If I have a fan blowing on me, within say 6' from my head, I will get an ear infection.

During the spring, summer and early fall, where I live gets to be blazing hot. This can be a dramatically difficult time for me, as I am more functional and generally a lot more capable when it is cool or cold outside. If the temperature in the room I'm trying to sleep in is close to 80 degrees or above, sleeping for me is very difficult. When my air conditioner is not working well, or it is just so hot that the air conditioner blowing at full force is not keeping my room at or below 80, it can be miserable trying to sleep. Once I manage to fall asleep, it seems I wake up fully every time I turn over or move, and it is not unusual to just have to get up for a while before trying to get back to sleep.

One of the biggest steps I've taken related for sleep hygiene to enhance my sleep involved buying a latex mattress and pillow. It was not a cheap purchase (am actually still paying on it) but one that has been very pleasant and worthwhile. It has really helped me sleep better, especially in the hotter periods of the year. Latex mattresses feel like memory foam mattresses, but natural latex (dunlop or talalay) has many strong benefits when it comes to health. For instance, they are naturally hypoallergenic, dust mite resistant and antimicrobial. Latex has small holes all throughout the mattress, which allows it to breathe and be cool when it is hot and warm when it is cold. As you may be able to tell, I highly recommend a natural latex mattress.

Daily Walking

Many walk multiple miles on their typical day. Some, more like myself, are sedentary, sitting a majority of their typical day. It is important for those who are like myself and very much sedentary, to take a walk daily. I am not sure whether I'd say standing for long periods is quite equivalent to walking, but it definitely is better than remaining in a seat all day.

For me, I think walking is actually easier than standing for long periods of time, as my joints can ache more while being still. Really, the more walking though the better. I try to shoot for at least 1 mile a day, and better yet 3 or more. For years I've walked to buy coffee each day, sometimes twice. The coffee shop has two locations, one is roughly a one mile walk in total (back and forth) and the second location is roughly a 3 mile walk in total (back and forth). Another thing I tend to do sometimes, even multiple times a day, is walk to one of the three grocery stores which are probably a quarter to half mile from my home. Something I enjoy a lot is hiking in the woods or just out in nature where there is open space and calm. I'm not as comfortable in public spaces or more so in crowds (like a mall).

Adding a daily walk will definitely benefit nearly any and/or everyone, unless there is another medical or physical matter which restricts one from being able to. Normally, I try to take the walk right after I've awoken and showered. Sometimes when I make my own coffee (which I've been doing more so lately), I have a harder time taking the walk, but it just depends on the day. As much as it is very difficult to wake up early in the day, in the morning, it seems to be becoming clearer (research-wise) that the earlier AM sun is the healthiest sun. Weather makes it a sort of seasonal thing, as with snow a walk is not necessarily inviting; and with the heat here in the summers, I can only take so much of one.

On the days that I do not take a walk I don't necessarily note it; but if I go for two or three days without having taken a walk, I definitely am able to note a more general lethargy.

Forever I've to some extent been involved in a physical activity, a sport, be it on and off, seasonally. In the summers I try to skate as much as I can, although I've slowed down a bit over these last few years from multiple times a week to multiple times a month. Hiking I enjoy, but the allergies can hit me hard; so I have to be very careful, because I have frequent headaches when I do much of it. Biking is similar to hiking for me, in that when I do a lot of it my allergies flare up, and/or additionally my shoulders along with neck will begin aching until it's a full blown headache/migraine. Sometimes it takes a motivating factor, like hunting morels or walking down to skate Homewoods (the concrete skate bowl that I helped to build nearly a mile down in deep woods, it is my good friend's bowl and property).

Not so often during the summers, I drive an hour to and then back, from where I can go to play ice hockey. If the city I live in would ever get its act together and keep the ice rink open year round, I would most definitely be playing at least once a week all year round. During the winter, I enjoy as much ice hockey as I can get and/or manage. Usually two games a week is just right, and often I want a third or fourth.

Some winters I get a fair amount of snowboarding in, which is not a lot, being 5-10 times total. Where I live, the ski/snowboard 'hill' is no mountain, so it is definitely not what it would be, where ideal. The 'hill' is an hour drive and has a vertical drop of 300 ft. This means you are on the lift a lot and the runs are over quick, no matter what you do. But, it is snowboarding, and I do enjoy it; so I can't really complain much.

Injuries – Toll Up (not a lifestyle adjustment)

With all of the intense sporting activities I've done so far in life, I've got a fair amount of aches and physical pains, and already quite frequently. It's all part of the game, so I cannot complain. Really, I'm stoked to still be able, to the extent which I am. Injury wise, I cannot begin to count but will attempt briefly mentioning a few of the more lingering ones. All through high school I had twists, sprains, scrapes, bruises, impacts, and swellings because I was skateboarding every single day, many days most of my free time. Also, I was attending ice hockey practices, as well as games, nearly daily through the winters. There'd been many injuries which kept me down or out for a brief while, a few that took me in to get checked out and a few that were quite scary. Something I feel is definitely not good, is the amount of times I've whip-lashed my neck...

The first bone I know that I broke was my right thumb at around 19 years old. Snowboarding on what was basically ice, as I carved (frontside) on my heel edge, I planted my hand forcefully on the ground behind me without being able to see it as I did it, but with my thumb basically pointing at the ice as it impacted. There was no fall but once I reached the base of the hill and was able to take off my glove, I was in much pain and it immediately looked really bad. There was blood from where my fingernail had been pressed upwards towards my wrist, puncturing my thumb. Worse than that though was the length of my thumb. It wasn't right and was very thick and short. It hurt a lot, and I ended up going to the hospital, arriving around two hours after it occurred. The doctor pulled it out and into place, saying there was a good chance I'd need later surgery involving a pin or pins. Thankfully, it healed up in the cast and I have not had issues with it what so ever. Taking notes at the time in college with my left hand (being right handed) was interesting, and I think actually was quite an awesome brain exercise to have done.

There was one minor head impact, thankfully wearing a helmet, while skateboarding at a park when I was 24 years old. Nothing more than feeling some discomfort occurred.

At 27 I took a really bad slam skateboarding. My right knee got bent wrong. As I carved out of a frontside (back facing the inside of the bowl, ledge or transition) grind on a steep 3' radius, 3' high transition, my back right foot slipped off of the tail, my knee folded, the shin and foot went upwards to the right towards my back right shoulder. There was a loud popping and I screamed loudly as it all happened. A couple of friends were skating at the park and they witnessed it. They both picked me up and escorted me to the hospital. It was a rough summer and doctors were difficult, in that they weren't giving me very detailed answers. That was until I sought a true knee specialist up in the state capital (an hour away) who was able to give me real answers. Six months later, in October 2007, I underwent a 'Patella Re-Alignment Surgery with Arthoscopy.' The surgery involved moving my lower patella tendon by cutting a slice of the shin bone where it meets the lower patella tendon, and then screwing it back in, but in the properly aligned (for the patella to move freely) spot. The arthroscope was used to clean the meniscus, trimming off broken, chipped cartilage. It was quite the ordeal, involving me having a machine, for two weeks after surgery, which continually bent my knee back and forth slowly in bed. Thankfully, I healed well and had no unfortunate mishaps. It was definitely the most serious surgery that I can, at least to an extent, recall going through. The screws, I had later removed, because I was having strange sensations upon impact in the area; they'd broken, so removal was good to have done.

At 29, I took a very, very bad fall skateboarding down a hill on my way to skate an indoor ramp. In hand was a cup of coffee. I was completely comfortable and confident going down the hill, I'd carved and power slid a couple of quick times, but I hit something and...

Regular footed is how I skate, which means my right foot is in the back and my left is in front, so imagine it as looking over your left shoulder going down the hill straight. It was near immediate, as I was scraping the back of my left shoulder all of a sudden as it hit the ground first, yet somehow my head was turned in a way that I was actually seeing over that same shoulder during the roll. Being so fast and hard of a fall, I cannot really fully understand how I contorted. In the end I was on my stomach and my wind was knocked out badly. I couldn't flip over easily but managed to quickly, out of a need to breathe. My left top to backside of shoulder, my upper back, my left hip, my right knee and both of my hands had road-rash bleeding scrapes. My two friends (one of whom had been at the skatepark two years earlier and had helped me to the hospital then) with whom I was meeting to skate the ramp, were already there and thankfully were still outside. They witnessed the fall and ran over immediately. Again this same friend drove me to the hospital. Now, I could go on and into what was one of the most horrific experiences of my life at the hospital that day; but I'll just say I was given no ice, while I was definitely stereotyped.

Regardless, the fall really messed me up and my spine will never be the same, as my left shoulder has always since felt slightly pushed forwards. Later, my friends who witnessed it told me that I had scorpioned (which means my feet came up and over my head behind me as I contorted into the ground). In the back of my mind, this fall may play directly into my 'Idiopathic Central Sleep Apnea' diagnosis/issue, in that the spinal cord relates to breathing. In the paperwork (that I had a hard time getting from the hospital years later) from the fall, there is quite a bit mentioned regarding cervical degenerative disease and specific damage in my cervical spine. So far, of the doctors I've spoken with, none have dove into this in any depth, and I have not been to a cervical spine specialist.

Just recently, snowboarding, I may have really injured my left knee from way too much impact. It is hard to say at this point and I am trying to baby it, slowly, to gauge in time whether or not I'm going to be able to proceed with my normal activities/routines...

Basic Routine Stretching / Exercises

A large piece of something that I do regularly, that I think helps me profoundly, is a routine. For two to three years now I've been doing this, anywhere from a few times a day to a handful of times each week. A series of stretches, basic exercises (you could say), involving slow repetitions of reaching upward and outwards, slowly counting and focusing on the body center or core. It is a bit tricky describing these clearly, but I will give it an attempt.

First, I bring my hands together pressing the palms and fingers together gently. While trying to keep my posture straight as I stand with my feet shoulder-width apart, upright, looking forwards with chin tucked and head up (gently pressed back). I try to locate the point of my center as I breathe in and out, positioning my hands pressed together in front of me, where they are comfortable and I am standing stable. This position I'll hold for 10 seconds, as I count slowly in my head. Then I reach upwards, keeping palms pressed gently together, lifting as far upwards as possible, with feet flat and stable, continuing to stand straight and still.

After this, I spread my arms straight out to my side, think of a T position. From there, I slowly bring my palms together, in front of me, 10 times slowly, always counting in my head as I go. Then I'll do the same but rather lifting my arms until my palms meet above my head, reaching and lifting as much as possible, but remaining stable and, of course, counting slowly. Then, I reach forwards with my arms straight, and I lift my stance onto my toes. This I hold sometimes for 10 seconds and sometimes for 30 seconds or longer. From there, I'll lift my arms as far upwards as I can reach, without standing on toes, and I'll hold for 10 seconds. Then, I lean forwards reaching down to my toes or the floor, and I'll hold for 10 seconds. I'll do a few sets of this.

Now, I do a set of exercises that are specifically meant for strengthening the muscles between the shoulder blades, a crucial muscle of the neck which helps one keep their head from falling or flailing around. As one gets older, their head will push or fall forwards more and more, this is something one really wants to avoid because as it happens the lower back and legs are affected very negatively. There is a lot that could be explained here, but I will rather just try to explain the exercise which was shown to me by an old high school friend, who for years worked as a physical therapist for a chiropractor. My friend told me that of all the exercises, this was really the one set that he felt was most valuable. So, begin as I described the T earlier, with both arms outwards to one's side while standing straight up, with chin tucked in and head gently pressed back, feet more or less shoulder width apart.

From here, very gently, just slightly reach straight backwards with both hands, focusing on squeezing the shoulder blades gently together and then go back to original position. Your arms don't need to move far, just a bit. Repeat this, doing it slowly, 10 times while counting and focusing on the shoulder blades squeezing together.

Now, lift arms above head and do the same motion, focusing on the same, 10 times.

Then, do the same while pointing downwards and outwards with arms, and imagine an upside down Y.

After this, lift the arms to be pointing upwards and outwards, like a Y, and do the same 10 repetitions while focusing.

Then, point towards toes and upwards slightly, and do the same, this time lifting the arms slightly as you lift, squeezing the shoulder blades together.

Not only should your focus be on gently squeezing the shoulder blades, but also on keeping your posture strong and straight, looking forwards and upwards but with chin tucked, head up.

Usually, I'll then lift a knee and hold my palms pressed gently together at center for 10 seconds. Then I'll lift hands with palms pressed together above my head as far as comfortably possible with knee still up and hold for 10 seconds.
From there, I'll reach outwards (like the T) and hold with knee up, for 10 seconds.
Finally, I'll then reach forwards with arms straight and will hold another 10 seconds. Sometimes I'll go back to palms together at center for a last 10 seconds.
After the one knee has been up, I'll then do the other knee up, same steps.
And to finish, I'll then do everything I've gone over, in reverse.

If it weren't for this set of stretches/exercises, I would not be doing the activities that I do. I feel very strongly that this routine for me is crucial to my overall stability and flexibility. It is both physically and mentally important.
This routine for me, can be seriously helpful and relieving when I'm not feeling necessarily well. There are days were I'm feeling aches and pains, maybe getting a headache, and by doing this simple routine, afterwards I always feel somewhat refreshed. Sometimes I'll actually feel free of, or released from, an oncoming headache. Yoga is a bit different, but I fully support it.
There is definitely something very valuable and real about meditation. I find the routine I've described for me to be meditative. Focusing only on my body while breathing and counting slowly, thinking on nothing, is grounding as well as somehow restorative.

Limit Stresses / Pressures / Anxieties

Obviously, this is something easier said than done. But it is
definitely something to consider and attempt to achieve. Doing so
for myself has been of crucial benefits. Doing so is not easy and will
be done differently for each one of us, all depending on the different
circumstances across the board. Here, I am very much speaking
directly at living having Narcolepsy with Cataplexy. Why? Well,
when you have Cataplexy that causes you to collapse, there are
serious risks. Besides physical risks, some may not even be
physical, but rather are mentally deep and sharp. Unfortunately,
this is all very complicated. But when you have a condition where
simple pleasures can trigger nearly instantly, complete temporary
paralysis, you learn (kind of by force) that you must be careful. To
be careful involves not putting yourself in obvious and/or clear
danger/s. Specific clear examples for me of what is seriously
physically risky, involve perhaps whether or not I should ride on a
roller coaster today (they are so fun, would it trigger Cataplexy?),
attempting to surf (would the possibility of pleasure from my first
successful run trigger Cataplexy in the water?). Skateboarding,
snowboarding, and playing ice hockey are things I know how to do
and things that I enjoy profoundly. They are things I'm not willing
to walk away from and, thankfully, can still manage to do. A sort of
less specific, but seriously broad example of what may be perhaps
mentally dangerous, would be simply joking around with someone
that I do not know well, cracking jokes with them. This may be
obvious, or maybe not. Above I stated, "with someone that I do not
know well," because it is a very real factor.

The reason I went into the above details or depth is because
Cataplexy for me has been something that will happen more often,
not only once it's already occurred, but also when there are any
more than the normal stresses, pressures or anxieties. It is very

hard to express the deepness that revolves around Cataplexy flaring up and/or being present. Cataplexy is something that is very different for each person who experiences it. So everything I say about it is from my own experience, though I have read descriptions of many others' experiences. There is a common theme with it though, which seems to be that there is no real predictability of Cataplexy nor manner of avoiding and/or ridding it entirely. And with regards to the triggers (or what the specific triggers are), for each person they are always different, varying. One major thing is, though, that Cataplexy escalates with escalation of overall stresses, pressures, or anxieties. It should also be noted, that all other symptoms of Narcolepsy escalate as well, with such...

Learn / Reflect / Understand / Appreciate

Upon confirmation of having Narcolepsy with Cataplexy, but more so upon learning more and more about what the disease is, it became very clear that I had to limit as much as I possibly could any and all stresses, pressures and/or anxieties. Doing so really required that I reflect upon myself, my place and surroundings, upon how I live, what I do, who I am around, where I go, when I do things, etc.

Very much I had to sort of put my foot down and walk away from certain things, or maybe I should say re-analyze my footing upon certain steps. A big part of that was researching and learning, attempting to grasp as best as I possibly could what the disease Narcolepsy with Cataplexy is.

Do not hesitate to ask your doctors what they think is occurring in the disease. It is worth confirming that they have an understanding, as they are there to help you (which, unfortunately, I've not always felt happens, due to constraints relating to it being part of what is, business).

Reading and participating on forums has been hugely helpful. It allowed me to learn not only what others go through themselves, but also how they deal with it and what helps them or doesn't help them. Reading medical research articles also was hugely helpful for learning about the specifics of what seems to be occurring, how the brain, the autoimmune and endocrine systems are involved.

I reflect continually and/or regularly, attempting to have solid footing or understanding of what it is I'm living with, not to mention trying to have awareness of what it is others may likely expect or think in regards to what it is that I'm living with.

By better understanding the disease, one is better able to explain to others and/or express what is occurring. Whether another will interpret and/or understand what is being said properly is another matter. Having a solid understanding of the disease will also help one to better juggle the symptoms.

It is important to form your own understanding, taking in what you can but double checking or confirming to the extent possible whether or not the connections fit accordingly. All too often, persons are expected to fit within, to follow the routine, to listen and be told so called information as if it is factual; when in reality we live in a constantly evolving and morphing realm, of so many variables that it is and will always remain impossible for any one alone, nor many combined, to actually know all that there is to know.

Don't assume there's always an easy route and/or a magical cure all which actually exist, and especially don't expect any such thing to be simply at your fingertips. What I'm really trying to say here is, be sure to think for yourself, seek confirmations and contemplate the things that matter to you. Simply put, be conscious.

Always, I've been one to observe, to prefer some sort of safe approach as well as safe exit over eagerness, lack of caution. Always thinking of others at least as much as of my own, and often perhaps thinking more for others than for my own.

Skateboarding, Nicaragua, private and public schools, the city within the region within the country and so on, my parents and family, my Brother and step-Father, learning and playing music, participating in team sports, traveling on my own often, learning and speaking a 2nd language, the many different friends and sorts of friends that I've had, just experiencing all that I have up to this point has definitely been wonderful and fascinating. The path you take, is more of a path you end up on, which isn't to say the path is set nor laid out, but is to say sometimes the path you end up on is far from what you could have ever previously envisioned; the path can go up and down, as the path goes on, on and possibly beyond...

Lifestyle Adjustments Recap

- Allergies Seasonal / Perennial -

Learn what you are allergic to and try to eventually figure out how the reactions affect you. Then do what you can to avoid and limit being exposed. If you are not suffering from allergies in some way and/or manner, then you are very lucky, and especially so, if you have Narcolepsy with Cataplexy.

- Food Allergies / Sensitivities -

Similarly to seasonal / perennial, learn what affects you and eventually how specifically. Take time and focus on eliminating the foods that trigger reactions. This is not easy for most and is a difficult but important path. Stay strong and be open to foods you may not have yet discovered or perhaps at some point previously didn't enjoy.

- Foods, Shopping, Balancing & Cooking-

As you must incorporate your food allergies plus sensitivities, you must incorporate elements of how you live and what you can manage to do, to find the right balance/s.

Be selective in what ingredients and what qualities as well as types of food that you choose to buy, cook with, and eat. Find what techniques work for you when it comes to cooking.

Pay close attention to what, where and how you eat, because if you don't, then it may be hard to note that something is negatively balanced, possibly bottle necking or disrupting something else, and maybe within such there's a simple fix to the balance.

Remember that food is the best medicine.

- Sleep Hygiene -
Routine, schedule, bed comfort, darkness, quietness, proper
temperature, naps, etc.
Do what you can to enhance your sleep hygiene. There are many
parts to it, some more important than others. Yet each part is
important for attempting to get the best sleep possible. Narcolepsy
causes difficulties with both sleeping well and having to sleep often
or somewhat sporadically. Being as comfortable as possible is of
importance (at least in my opinion).

- Daily Walking -
1 mile + per day and preferably, more.
Unless you already walk or perhaps stand lots every day, then
make walking a part of your daily routine. Such will help your
overall health.
The 'Center for Advancing Health' says that less than a ¼ of
Americans walk for more than 10 minutes a week...

- Basic Routine Stretching / Exercise -
A routine explained. One that I do daily, sometimes multiple times.

- Limit Stresses / Pressures / Anxieties -
Not going to be simple, easy, nor universal. Regardless, important.

- Learn / Reflect / Understand / Appreciate -
Dive in deeply, observe with focus, take in what you can, and then
contemplate upon it. Stir up your own perspective with trying
others'. Look for reflections and connections, be it relating to
Narcolepsy with Cataplexy or whatever, and so much more.
Let the world, the tech, the times and people fascinate you..!

Expressions of My Own 'Narcolepsy with Cataplexy': An onwards roller coaster ride it is...

Above is a book that I (Narcoplexic) published in October, 2013; available online from Amazon, or the CreateSpace Store.

The title is exactly what it is, my own expressions.
-Sketches/Illustrations along with many descriptions, going into my experience/s living, having Narcolepsy with Cataplexy.
-There is detailed, factual information on Narcolepsy with or without Cataplexy.
-Many of the points that I attempt to hit on, express, and convey within it, are very misunderstood, touching on each of the 4 tetrad symptoms, in detail, of Narcolepsy with or without Cataplexy...
-Gets into deep specifics on the difficulties, and certain unique occurrences, as well as thoughts of my own, all relating to the disease.

What's to come next? I am not sure.
There's a whole lot that I didn't go into, as far as myself and my past.
Maybe and likely so, I'll feel like diving into more, at a later point?
Nicaragua was hardly mentioned and it is, the people are, so much a part of my roots and perspectives. There's many medical interactions, experiences that have just been profoundly difficult and painful. Speaking of social limitations and/or difficulties, ordeals to do with interpersonal relations, communications. There's a time and place though, for what comes; and especially when in regards to Narcolepsy with Cataplexy.

Skateparks, and related advocacy, are hugely important in my eyes and possible/likely things that I'll do some writing on, in depth eventually...
Find some of my 3D Rhinoceros, Skatepark Conceptual Design Renderings at: www.HungerSkateparks.com
[Support your local Skaters, & Skateparks built by Skater/Builders]

['Thank You']
Narcoplexic@Narcoplexic.com
Facebook.com/Narcoplexic
youtube.com/RightTrash